ENT TZAR

Ear Nose and Throat for Medical Students

A case-based approach

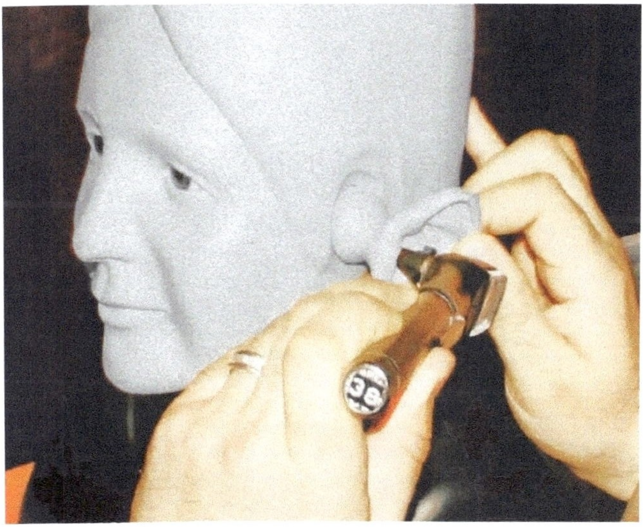

Ricardo Persaud | Sridhayan Mahalingam
Alexander Yao | Shradha Gupta | Ruchir Singh

Foreword by **Professor Antony Narula** FRCS

Imperial College London Medical School, UK

1st Edition 2015

Ear Nose and Throat for Medical Students

A case-based approach

RICARDO AP PERSAUD
FRCS ORL-HNS (Eng), CCT Otol. (UK),
MBBS, MSB, CBiol, MPhil, MRCS (Gen), DO-HNS
Consultant ENT Head Neck & Facial Plastic Surgeon
Al Zahra Hospital, Sharjah, PO Box 3499, UAE
Former Examiner in Surgery, Imperial College Medical School
London, UK.

SRIDHAYAN MAHALINGAM
BSc (Hons), MBBS, MSc, MRCS (ENT), DO-HNS
Core Surgical Trainee, East Surrey Hospital, Redhill, UK.

ALEXANDER YAO
MBBS (Distinction), BA (Cantab)
Academic Foundation Doctor, Freeman Hospital
Newcastle Upon Tyne Hospitals NHS Trust
Training Fellow at Newcastle University, UK.

SHRADHA GUPTA
BSc (Hons), MBBS (Distinction), MRCS, DO-HNS
Specialist Registrar in Otolaryngology
Leicester Royal Infirmary, UK.

RUCHIR SINGH
BSc (Hons) MBChB (Hons)
Academic Foundation Doctor
Leicester, UK.

FastPrint Publishing

www.fast-print.net/store.php

EAR NOSE AND THROAT FOR MEDICAL STUDENTS:
A CASE-BASED APPROACH

A catalogue record for this book is available from the British Library

ISBN 978-178456-171-0

First published 2015 by Fast-Print Publishing, Peterborough, England.

Ear Nose and Throat for Medical Students:

A Case-Based Approach

CONTENTS

- Preface 7
- Foreword 9
- Acknowledgements 11
- Dedications 12
- Glossary 13

CHAPTER 1: BASICS **15**

1.1 History

1.1.1 History Taking 15

1.1.2 ENT Symptoms 17

1.2 Examinations

1.2.1 Ear 21

1.2.2 Nose 32

1.2.3 Oral cavity and Throat 36

1.2.4 Neck 39

1.2.5 Thyroid Status and related structures 45

1.3 Investigations

1.3.1 Pure Tone Audiogram 47

1.3.2 Tympanogram 51

1.3.3 Radiology: CT and MRI 53

CHAPTER 2: EAR **55**

2.1 Outer ear

2.1.1 External Ear trauma 55

2.1.2 Pinna Haematoma 59

2.1.3 Perichondritis 62

2.1.4 Otitis Externa 65

2.1.5 Foreign Body in the Ear 68

2.2 Middle ear
2.2.1 Perforation of Tympanic Membrane 71
2.2.2 Temporal Bone Fracture 74
2.2.3 Facial Nerve Palsy 79
2.2.4 Acute Otitis Media 81
2.2.5 Acute Mastoiditis 90
2.2.6 Eustachian Tube Dysfunction 93
2.2.7 Otitis Media with Effusion 97
2.2.8 Cholesteatoma 100
2.2.9 Presbyacusis 104
2.2.10 Noise-induced Hearing Loss 107
2.2.11 Otosclerosis 110
2.3 Inner ear
2.3.1 Benign Paroxysmal Positional Vertigo (BPPV) 113
2.3.2 Meniere's Disease 118
2.3.3 Labyrinthitis 122
2.3.4 Vestibular Schwannoma 127
2.3.5 Central Causes of Vertigo 130

CHAPTER 3: NOSE AND SINUSES 132
3.1 Nose
3.1.1 Nasal Trauma 132
3.1.2 Foreign Body in the Nose 137
3.1.3 Epistaxis 139
3.1.4 Septal Perforation and Granulomatous Disorders 144
3.1.5 Nasal Polyps 147
3.1.6 Rhinitis 151
3.1.7 Nasopharyngeal carcinoma 157
3.2 Sinuses
3.2.1 Rhinosinusitis 157
3.2.2 Periorbital Cellulitis 163
3.2.3 Sinonasal Malignancy 166

CHAPTER 4: HEAD, NECK AND THROAT **169**

4.1 Infective

4.1.1 Tonsillitis 169

4.1.2 Superficial Neck Abscess 173

4.1.3 Deep Neck Space Infections 175

4.1.4 Head and Neck Tuberculosis 178

4.2 Non-Infective

4.2.1 Airway Obstruction 182

4.2.2 Gastro-oesophageal reflux disease (GORD) and laryngopharyngeal reflux (LPR) 188

4.2.3 Pharyngeal Pouch 191

4.2.4 Voice Disorders 195

4.2.5 Benign Salivary gland disease 199

4.2.6 Thyroid Disease (Benign and Malignant) 203

4.2.7 Laryngeal malignancy 213

4.3 Surgical Procedures

4.3.1 Tracheostomies 216

4.3.2 Laryngectomy 219

4.3.3 Reconstruction in the Head and Neck 222

CHAPTER 5: PAEDIATRIC OTOLARYNGOLOGY **225**

5.1 Congenital Abnormalities

5.1.1 Congenital Abnormalities of Ears and Hearing 225

5.1.2 Congenital Abnormalities of the Nose 229

5.1.3 Congenital Abnormalities: Cleft Conditions 231

5.1.4 Congenital Abnormalities of The Neck 233

5.2 Genetic Syndromes

5.2.1 Down's Syndrome and ENT 237

5.2.2 Other Syndromes and ENT 238

5.3 Paediatric Airways

5.3.1 Paediatric Airway Issues 240

5.3.2 Obstructive Sleep Apnoea 247

PREFACE

Ear, Nose and Throat for Medical Students is a new and innovative book that provides a myriad of common case presentations to guide your learning. The impetus for writing this book came from the feedback received from medical students in various UK medical schools.

The book covers common ear, nose and throat conditions that can be seen in daily practice and incorporates aspects of head and neck surgery and paediatric otolaryngology. It also offers detailed approaches to history taking, examination and investigation interpretation.

Each fictional case is introduced by a brief history, followed by questions regarding diagnostic reasoning, management and viva questions. The mixed format of clinical cases and basic science helps the reader to improve their clinical skills as well as reinforce their understanding of key pathophysiology.

The colourful and concise layout of the text with relevant pictures help to facilitate your learning, increase your confidence in otolaryngology and make studying an enjoyable experience.

Whilst this book is primarily aimed at medical students worldwide, it may also be useful to interns and even general practitioners who see ENT related conditions. It is designed to be used as an *aid* to both the written and OSCE final examinations. The management and approach of many conditions will vary with time and location; hence this book is not intended to be didactic and should not replace medical teaching, local hospital protocols or textbooks.

Mr Ricardo Persaud is a Consultant ENT Surgeon who has vast experience of Otolaryngology and written several successful books. Contributions from his trainee colleagues have ensured that this book is both approachable and appropriate for your learning. We hope this book is just as enjoyable to read as it was to produce.

Ricardo AP Persaud
Sridhayan Mahalingam
Alexander Yao
Shradha Gupta
Ruchir Singh

January 2015

FOREWORD

It gives me great pleasure to write the foreword for *Ear Nose and Throat for Medical Students*, which is written by a team of British-trained doctors. From the content and presentation of this book, it is clear that a great deal of thought, time, effort and devotion has been spent on the project. After carefully reading through the content, I strongly believe the authors have achieved their main aim of providing a solid understanding of key issues pertaining to undergraduate ENT training, including the basic elements of history taking, examination and investigations. This is particularly important as only little time is devoted to ENT in most medical school curriculum worldwide.

The case-based format of the book is an excellent way of providing a good understanding of the pathway from presentation to treatment. Furthermore, it encourages learning as well as the application of knowledge in a clinical and relevant manner. This book also contains invaluable tips and tricks, which could make that crucial difference in your written and OSCE examinations. I have no doubt that *Ear Nose and Throat for Medical Students* will be popular among medical students around the world, and even General Practitioners, because of its content validity and the simple clear presentation of the essential information relevant to Otolaryngology.

Professor Antony Narula MA FRCS FRCS Ed
Examiner Imperial College London Medical School
Consultant ENT Surgeon, Imperial College Hospitals (St Mary's Hospital)
Visiting Professor, Middlesex University
Council Member Royal College of Surgeons of England
Past President of British Society of Otology
Past Examiner FRCS ORL-HNS Intercollegiate Board
President-Elect ENT UK.

November 2014

ACKNOWLEDGMENTS

Many thanks to Dr Raunak Singh MBChB, Core Trainee, Leicester, UK for his comments and generous help with formatting the document and to all the medical students who suggested the key topics. We are also grateful to all our colleagues and patients who provided consent to appear in this book.

DEDICATIONS

To all the ambassadors of ENT TZAR
Past, Present and Future

GLOSSARY

AC – air conduction
ACE – Angiotensin converting enzyme
AF - Atrial fibrillation
ANCA – anti-neutrophil cytoplasmic antibody
ARS – acute rhinosinusitis
AOM – acute otitis media
BAHA – bone anchored hearing aid
BC – bone conduction
BIPP – bismuth iodoform paraffin paste
BPPV – benign paroxysmal positional vertigo
CHL – Conductive hearing loss
CN7/VII – 7th cranial nerve i.e. facial
CSF – cerebrospinal fluid
CT – computed tomography
CNS – central nervous system
CRP – C-reactive protein
CSOM – chronic suppurative otitis media
CST – cavernous sinus thrombosis
CSF- cerebrospinal fluid
CXR – chest x-ray
DH – drug history
EAC – external auditory canal
EUA – examination under anaesthesia
FBC – full blood count
FESS- functional endoscopic sinus surgery
FH- family history
FNA – fine needle aspiration
FNE – flexible nasendoscopy
G+S – group and save
GA – general anaesthetic
GCS – Glasgow Coma Scale
GORD – gastro-oesophageal reflux disease
HHT – hereditary haemorrhagic telangiectasia

Hx - history
ICP – intracranial pressure
I&D – incision and drainage
IM - intramuscular
INR – international normalised ratio
IV – intravenous
Ix - investigations
LMN – lower motor neurone
MC&S – microscopy culture and sensitivity
MDT – multidisciplinary team
MRI – magnetic resonance imaging
MS – multiple sclerosis
MUA – manipulation under anaesthesia
Mx - management
NBM – nil by mouth
O/E – on examination
OGD – oesophagogastroduodenoscopy
OPD – outpatient department
PC – presenting complaint
PMH- past medical history
PRN – *Pro re nata* (latin). 'As needed'
PTA – pure tone audiogram
RAST – radioallergosorbent test
SIGN – Scottish intercollegiate guidelines network
SNHL – sensorineural hearing loss
SSNHL – sudden sensorineural hearing loss
TM – tympanic membrane
U&Es – urea and electrolytes
UMN – upper motor neurone
URTI – upper respiratory tract infection
WCC – white cell count

Chapter 1

Basics

1.1 HISTORY

1.1.1 HISTORY TAKING

General Structure

- Presenting Complaint
- History of Presenting Complaint
    - Timing: Onset, duration, fluctuation, progression, number of events?
    - Quality and Description of symptom: character, severity, aggravating or relieving factors, does it affect daily life?
- Past Medical History
- Drug History and Allergies
- Family History
- Social History: ask about relevant risk factors, occupation, age, smoking and alcohol intake, who do they live with? Are they worried about anything in particular because of this?

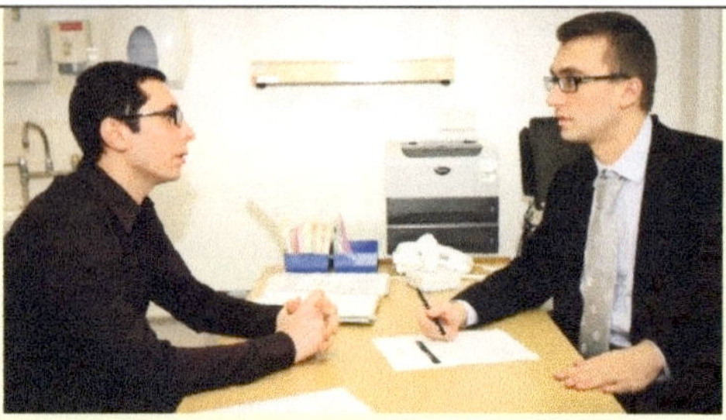

Figure 1.1.1a Formal set up for history taking (with a table barrier)

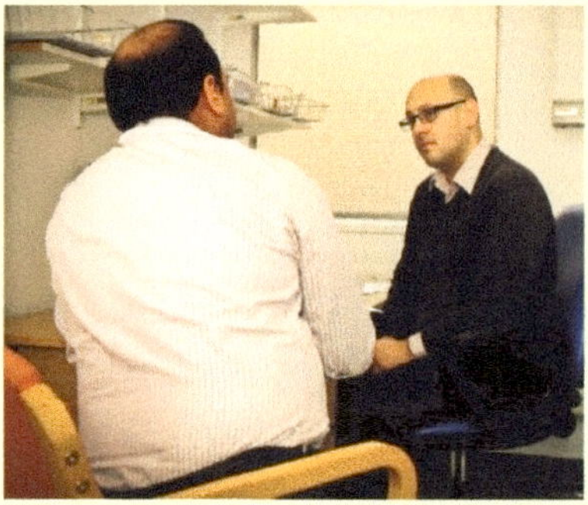

Figure 1.1.1b. Less formal arrangement for history taking (without a table barrier)

1.1.2 ENT SYMPTOMS

Anatomical region	Symptoms	Differentials
Ear (HOPES)	**H**earing loss	Conductive (wax, otitis media ± effusion, tympanic membrane pathology, otosclerosis) Sensorineural (noise induced, infective, genetic, presbyacusis, vestibular schwannoma, Meniere's)
	Otorrhoea	Otitis media with perforation, foreign body, CSF otorrhoea, otitis externa
	Pain	Acute otitis externa/media, Ramsay Hunt Syndrome, referred pain from nose or throat.

	Equilibrium (balance/dizziness/vertigo)	BPPV, Meniere's, vestibular neuritis, labyrinthitis, M.S, vestibular schwannoma, migraine, drug induced
	Sounds (tinnitus)	Wax, otosclerosis, Meniere's, loud noises, hypertension, drug induced
Nose (ROPES)	**R**hinorrhoea	Rhinitis, foreign body, epistaxis, CSF rhinorrhoea
	Obstruction	Genetic or structural deformity, foreign body, rhinitis, polyps, septal deviation, sinusitis, tumours
	Pain or pressure	Sinusitis, migraines, trigeminal neuralgia, dental causes e.g. abscess
	Epistaxis	Idiopathic, trauma, neoplastic, rhinitis, hereditary coagulopathies, systemic disease e.g. hypertension, anticoagulants

	Sense of smell	Traumatic head injury, respiratory tract infections, nasal obstruction, nerve damage
Throat (SWOT BDS)	**S**wellings or Lumps	Thyroid lumps, pharyngeal pouch, salivary gland lumps, lymph nodes, carotid body aneurysm or tumour, cystic hygroma
	Weight loss	Malignancy, difficulty swallowing, chronic inflammation.
	Odynophagia/dysphagia	Infective, inflammatory, infiltrative lesions.
	Temperature	Inflammatory, infective. Some malignancies.
	Blood	From larynx, pharynx, lungs, oesophagus.

	Dysphonia	Laryngitis, vocal cord nodules, respiratory tract infections, carcinoma, smoking, GORD, recurrent laryngeal nerve palsy, congenital, neurological disease
	Sweating	Sweating is a 'B' symptom relevant to lymphoma

1.2 EXAMINATIONS

1.2.1 EAR

Introduction

- Introduce yourself
- Obtain name, age
- Gain consent
- Wash hands
- Ask patient which is their better hearing ear
- Check whether there is any pain before starting

Inspection

Inspect the patient from the front, checking for any asymmetry. Closely inspect the better ear first:

- Check the pinna. Comment on any abnormalities in shape, size or developmental structural abnormalities
- Check behind and above the ear for scars
- Inspect mastoid area for any swelling or erythema
- Check the pre-auricular area for scars or a pre-auricular sinus

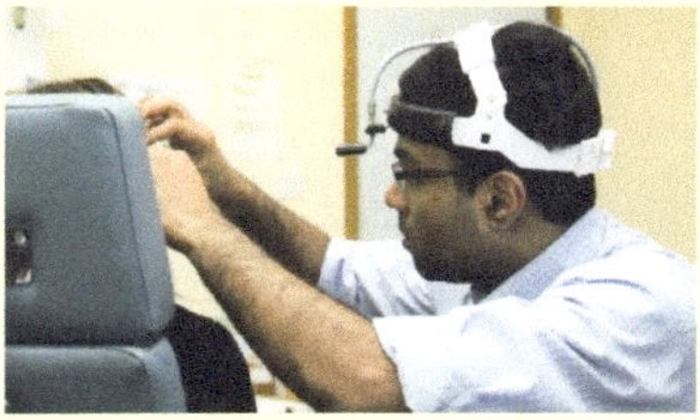

Figure 1.2.1. Inspection of the ear – note the use of head light and the doctor is sititng comfortable at the same level as the patient

Otoscopy

- In adults the pinna should be pulled up and backwards
- In children the pinna should be pulled down and backwards
- Gently insert the otoscope into the ear
- Carefully examine the external auditory canal
- Examine the tympanic membrane using the 4 question **MIPC** method:
    - **M** – where is the **M**alleus? (identification of the malleus is assurance that you are looking at the tympanic membrane)
    - **I** –drum **I**ntact (i.e. is there a perforation in the pars tensa or pars flaccida)?
    - **P** –**P**osition of the tympanic membrane (normal, retracted or bulging)?
    - **C** –**C**olour of the tympanic membrane (grey, dull, pink, white, blue etc)
- Change the speculum. This prevents transmission of infection.
- Inspect and Examine the OPPOSITE ear in a similar manner

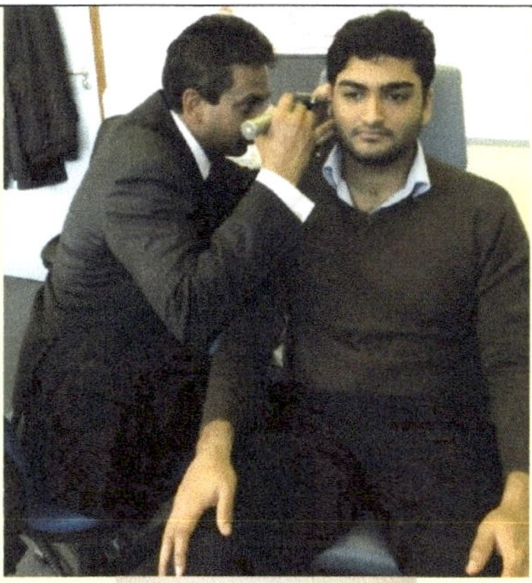

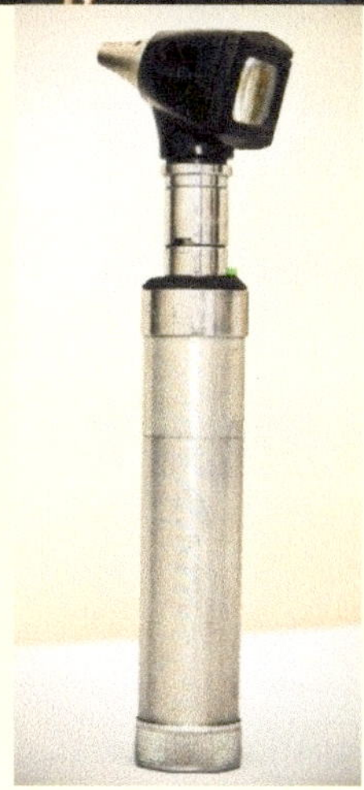

Figures 1.2.1a and 1.2.1b Correct position to examine the ear with an auroscope, i.e., sit comfortably so that you are at the same level as the patient (note the correct way to hold the auroscope). A typical auroscope is shown in Fig 1.2.1b.

Useful Tip

- The auroscope should be held like a pen
- Attach a disposable aural speculum to the end
- Hold the auroscope in the same hand as the ear being examined i.e. right hand for right ear and left hand for left ear
- Rest the little finger of the hand against the patient's cheek gently for stability, and prevent ear injury in case the patient jerks. This is especially important in children.
- Use the opposite hand to pull the pinna into position

Tuning Fork Tests

As part of the ear examination you may be expected to perform a basic tuning fork test to check for sensorineural or conductive hearing loss.

- The Weber test detects a difference in hearing between the two ears.
- The Rinne test can **confirm** presence of CHL since the Weber test only detects a difference of hearing between the two ears.
- Use a 512Hz tuning fork
- Strike the tines of the fork firmly against your elbow/knee for adequate vibration

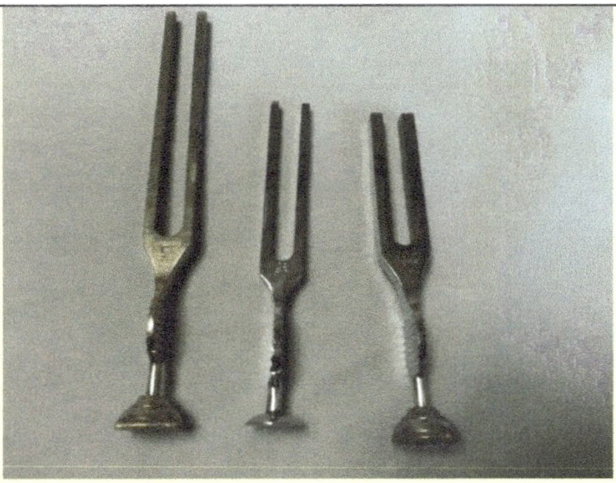

Figure 1.2.1c Tuning forks. Make sure you use the most appropriate one (512Hz)

WEBER'S Test

- Activate the tuning fork as described
- Place the base of the fork in the centre of the patient's forehead or on the top of the patient's head
- Ask where the sound is loudest – right ear, left ear or in the middle?

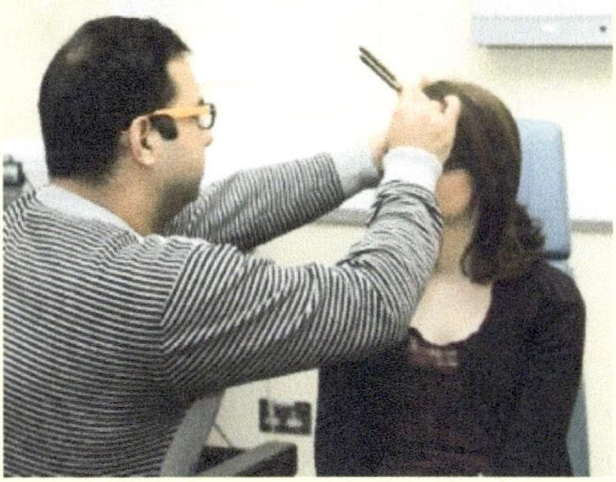

Figure 1.2.1c Weber test

Interpret results:

- Normal hearing – Sound is central
- Sensorineural hearing loss – Sound heard loudest in contralateral ear
- Conductive hearing loss – Sound heard loudest in ipsilateral ear.

RINNE'S Test

- Activate the tuning fork as described
- Hold the fork against the mastoid process. (This is position 1)
- Next move the fork in front of the patient's ear. The tines should be held parallel and 2 cm away from the external auditory meatus. (This is position 2)
- Ask the patient "which sound is louder? Position 1 or 2?"

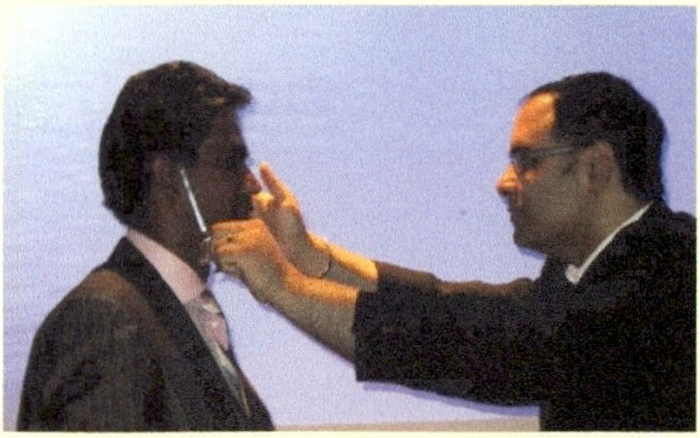

Figure 1.2.1d Rinne test

Interpret results:

- The test compares air conduction (AC) with bone conduction (BC). Remember that normally air conduction should be superior to bone conduction i.e. the sound should be heard loudest in front of the ear (position 2).
- Rinne Positive: Air conduction is better than bone conduction
- Rinne Negative: Bone conduction is better than air conduction

Tuning Fork Reference Tables

	Weber lateralises left	**Weber lateralises right**
Rinne positive both ears **AC>BC**	SNHL in right	SNHL in left
Rinne negative left **BC >AC**	Conductive loss in left	SNHL in left
Rinne negative right **BC>AC**	SNHL in right	Conductive loss in right

	Normal	**CHL**	**SNHL**
Weber	Midline	Lateralises to affected ear	Lateralises to better ear
Rinne	Positive (AC>BC)	Negative (BC>AC)	Positive (AC>BC)

Free Field Vocal Test and Interpretation

Method

- Choose a letter and number combination e.g. A1
- Position yourself in line with the side being tested
- Mask the other ear using the tragal rub technique
- Start by whispering the combination at 60cm
- Ask the patient to repeat the combination
- If they cannot repeat the combination step-up in sound level to conversational voice at 60cm and then to a loud voice at 60cm then 15cm.
- Stop when they can repeat the combination correctly >50% of the time

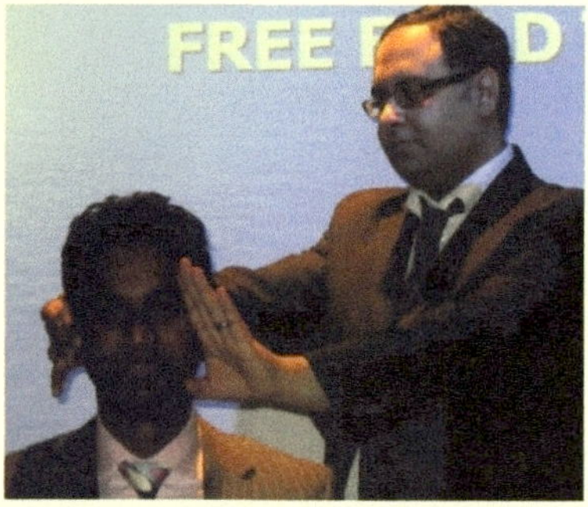

Figure 1.2.1d. Free field testing

Interpretation

- Can hear whisper at 60cm
    - Normal hearing (< 30dBHL)
- Can hear conversational voice at 60cm
    - Mild / moderate loss (30-60dBHL)
- Can hear loud voice at 60cm
    - Moderate / severe loss (60-90dBHL)

- Can only hear loud voice at 15cm
    - Profound loss (>90dBHL)

Fistula Test

This is designed to test for a perilymphatic fistula.

- Apply positive pressure to the tympanic membrane by applying pressure to the tragus for a few seconds
- The presence of a fistula in the examined ear will produce nystagmus
- Nystagmus will occur towards the affected ear

Facial Nerve Examination

The branches of the facial nerve should be examined as part of the full ear exam as it can be affected by otological pathology during its course through the temporal bone or middle ear.

Ask the patient to:

- Raise their eyebrows (Temporal Branch)
- Close their eyes tightly (Zygomatic Branch)
- Blow out the cheeks (Buccal Branch)
- Smile (Marginal Mandibular Branch)
- Tense the neck (or grimace) (Cervical Branch)

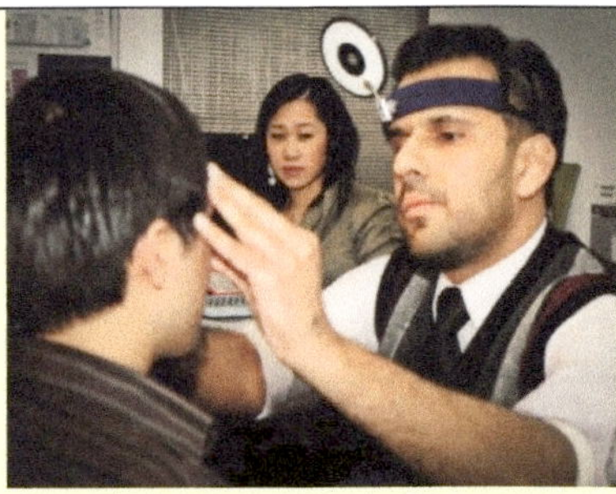

Figure 1.2.1e Facial nerve examination (opening the eyes against resistance – tempero-zygomatic branches of the facial nerve)

Completing the Examination
• Thank the patient • Wash your hands • Summarise your findings

Additional Tests
• Flexible nasendoscopy to rule out nasopharyngeal mass obstructing Eustachian Tube • Pure Tone Audiometry • Tympanogram

Advanced Tips

- Remove glasses before examining the ear
- Check in the hairline for scars from mastoid surgery
- Check the scalp for the presence of a Bone Anchored Hearing Aid (BAHA)
- Remove hearing aid/BAHA when testing hearing but remember to give the instructions first whilst the hearing aid is in place and then ask patient to remove it!

1.2.2 NOSE

Introduction

- Introduce yourself
- Obtain name, age
- Gain consent
- Wash hands
- Ask about any pain before starting
- Prepare yourself e.g. equipment (headlight), seating position

Inspection

Generally inspect for:

- Symmetry
- Scars or signs of recent operation/trauma?
- Erythema
- Dorsal hump, tip ptosis, saddle deformity, lateral deviation. Observe these from front, side, and if possible from the top (as the patient reclines on the couch)

Now inspect locally:

- Lift nasal tip: Assess vestibule and caudal end of septum
- Anterior rhinoscopy: Using Thudicum's speculum look for the following features
    - Septal deviation
    - Septal perforation
    - Nasal mucosa changes
    - Turbinates
    - Polyps

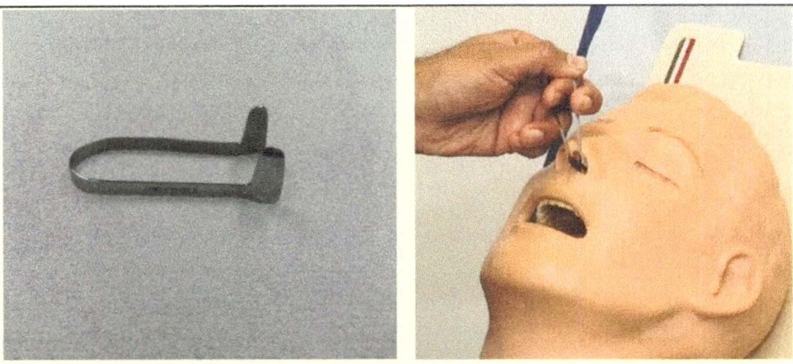

Figure 1.2.2a-b Thudicum Speculum used for anterior rhinoscopy and the correct way to hold it.

Function

• Patency of nasal airway:
    o Inflow: look for alar collapse
    o Outflow: check misting size and pattern on a cold Lack's tongue depressor
• Olfactory function:
    o Ask about sense of smell
    o Olfactory testing kit

Flexible Nasendoscopy

This is an essential part of upper airway examination from the nose to the larynx and it is performed routinely by ENT Surgeons. Training is required to use a flexible nasendoscope and to identify the following:

- Posterior septum
- Turbinates
- Nasopharynx, adenoidal pad
- Eustachian tube orifices
- Fossa of Rosenmüller. Nasopharyngeal cancers here can cause Eustachian tube obstruction and hence middle ear pathology.

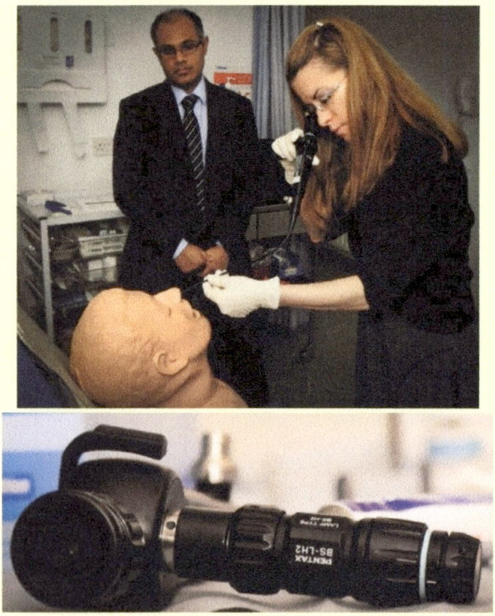

Figure 1.2.2c. Flexible Nasendoscopy with portable light source attached

Neck

- Palpate neck for any lumps or lymphadenopathy (submandibular, deep cervical)

Completing the Examination

- Thank the patient
- Wash your hands
- Summarise your findings

1.2.3 ORAL CAVITY AND THROAT

Introduction

- Introduce yourself
- Obtain name, age
- Gain consent
- Wash hands
- Ask about any pain before starting
- Prepare yourself e.g. equipment (headlight), seating position

Inspection

- Symmetry, scars, erythema, tracheostomy?
- Examine oral cavity using two tongue depressors, identify and comment on
    - Buccal mucosa
    - Stensen's (parotid) duct
    - Floor of mouth
    - Wharton's duct (submandibular)
    - Dentition, gums.
- Inspect the tonsils, uvula, posterior pharyngeal wall

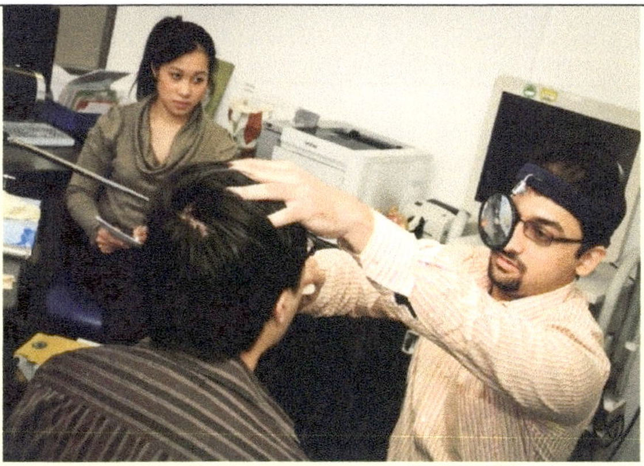

Figure 1.2.3 Oral examination using head mirror and tongue depressor

Palpation
• Bimanual palpation of the salivary glands (parotid and submandibular). Describe any changes or lumps that can be felt. These may be tumours or stones.

Flexible Nasendoscopy

If trained, use this to look for the following structures, noting any abnormalities

- Post-nasal space
- Base of tongue
- Epiglottis
- Valleculae
- Larynx
- Vocal cords
- Arytenoids
- Ventricular folds
- Piriform fossae

Speech

- Ask patient to count to ten
- Assess for any hoarseness or 'breathy' speech

Completing the Examination

- Thank the patient
- Wash your hands
- Summarise your findings

1.2.4 NECK

Introduction

- Introduce yourself, gain consent, and wash hands.
- Obtain the name, age
- Exposure– ask them to unbutton their shirt as appropriate
- Positioning- Ask to move forward from wall as appropriate (as you will need to go behind patient to examine their neck.
- Make sure you are clear whether you have been asked to examine (just) the neck lump or also thyroid status (also a common exam topic).

Inspection

- General inspection: clothes, hot and sweaty, note their voice, signs of weight loss or gain.

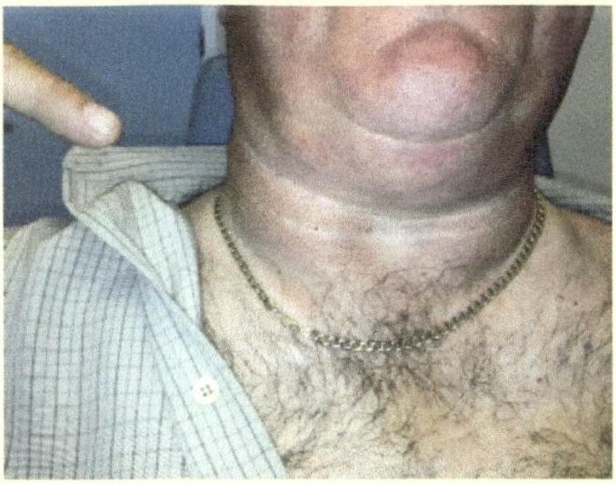

Figure 1.2.4 The patient may help you to identify the problem as shown here (large goitre)

Palpation of Neck/lumps

Neck – from the front

- Inspect for lumps. Note the characteristics as for any lump. Don't forget to transilluminate. (Transillumination suggests a cystic nature.)

Then ask patient to:

- Sip water: Watch movement of lump superiorly with swallowing. This suggests thyroid origin.
- Stick out tongue: If tongue moves up, this suggests a possible thyroglossal cyst.

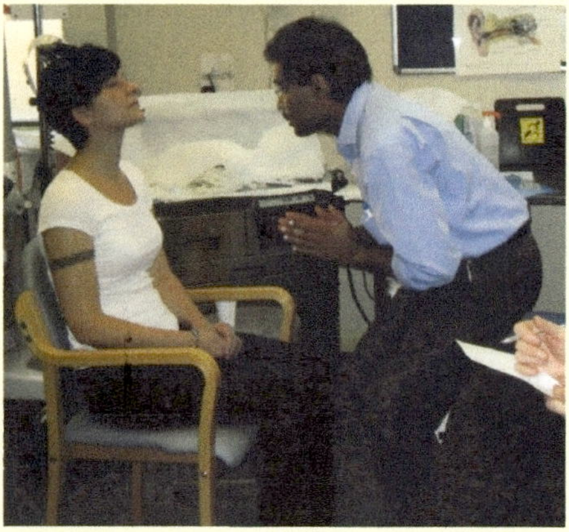

Figure 1.2.4a A candidate carefully inspecting the neck

Neck – from the side

- Look in profile at eyes– proptosis.
- Look in profile at lump. Consider asking to swallow again if it was unclear on inspection from the front.

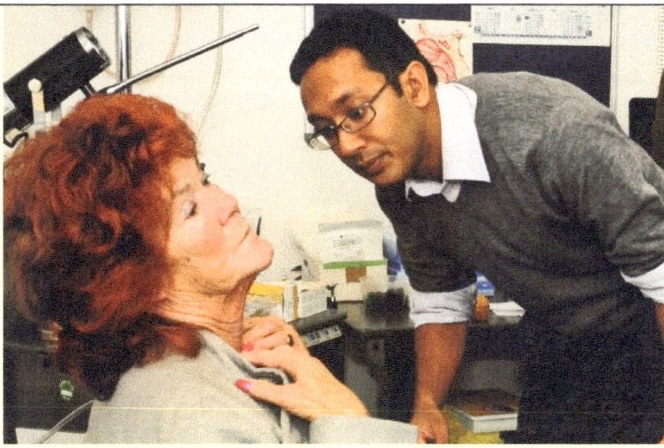

Figure 1.2.4b Inspection from the side

Neck – standing behind the patient

- Tell the patient you are going to examine their neck by standing behind them.
- Identify the thyroid/neck lump, and note its features. E.g. nodular, smooth, etc.
- Ask patient to swallow
- Ask patient to stick out tongue

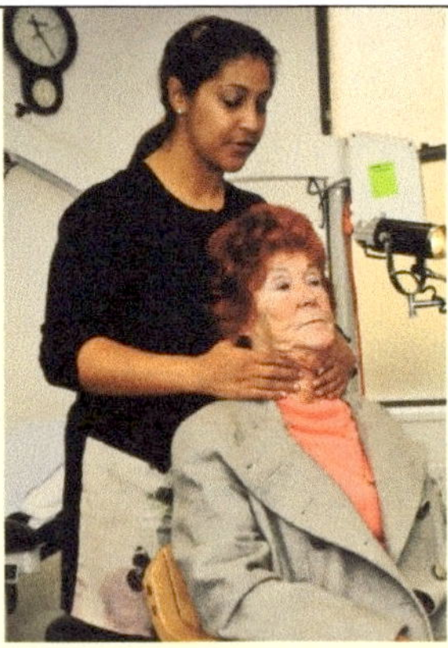

Figure 1.2.4c Correction position for palpation of the neck

Completing the Examination

- Whilst still standing behind the patient, examine the neck lymph nodes systematically.
- Auscultate for bruits. May be present in hyperthyroidism.
- Percuss for retrosternal extension of goitre.
- Ask patient to raise both their arms above their head to elicit 'Pemberton's sign'. Large retrosternal goitres may cause thoracic outlet obstruction, compressing the SVC and disrupting venous return. Facial flushing, distended neck veins, elevated JVP are all possible features of this sign.

Useful Tips

How to Describe a Neck lump:

When describing a neck lump, it is important to note and examine for the following features - **'St Face Rim':**

- **S**
  - Site
  - Size
  - Shape
  - Surface
  - Skin/scars
- **T**
  - Temperature
  - Tender
  - Transilluminate

Examination of the Lymph nodes:

One method to systematically examine the lymph nodes:

- Start at pre-tracheal nodes.
- Submental. Then move along jaw.
- Submandibular.
- Jugulodigastric lymph nodes.
- Pre-auricular.
- Post-auricular.

Then describe other important features where appropriate:

- **F**. Fixed.
- **A.** Attachment.
- **C.** Consistency
- **E**. Expansile (e.g. arterial source)

- **R**. Reducible. (possible hernias)
- **I**. Irreducible. (possible hernias)
- **M**. Mobile.

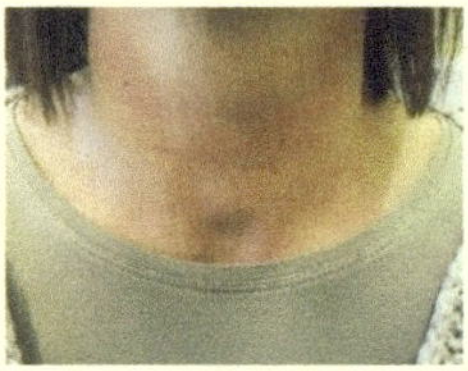

Figure 1.2.4d Neck lump in the thyroid isthmus

- Anterior cervical chain. Moving down the anterior border of the sternocleidomastoid.
- Supraclavicular.
- Posterior cervical chain. Moving up the anterior border of the upper trapezius.
- Occipital.

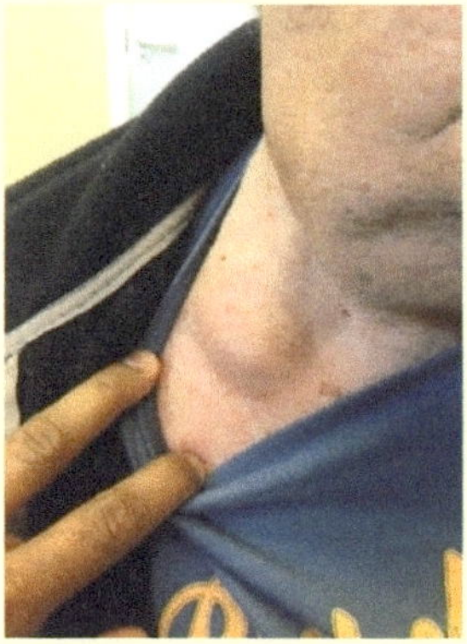

Figure 1.2.4e Cervical lymphadenopathy

1.2.5 THYROID STATUS AND RELATED STRUCTURES

Introduction

- Introduce yourself, gain consent, and wash hands.
- Obtain the name, age and occupation of the patient
- Ask to expose– ask them to unbutton their shirt as appropriate

Head

- Work from top to bottom not missing any key steps- use anatomy as landmarks.
- Eyebrows - thinning? Loss of outer thirds in hypothyroidism.
- Eyes
    - Make sure you examine eye movement and lid lag.
    - Looking for 4 features: exophthalmos, proptosis, ophthalmoplegia, and lid lag– all features of hyperthyroidism.

Hands and Arms

- Hands - start at nails and move proximally.
    - Acropachy/onycholysis etc.
- Palms - palmar erythema, sweaty, cold. Pale palmar creases indicating anaemia in hypothyroidism.
- Paper on the outstretched hands – test for fine tremor
- Wrist
    - Pulse – AF in hyperthyroidism, bradycardia in hypothyroidism
    - Carpal tunnel scars– carpal tunnel syndrome is associated with hypothyroidism

Additional Tests and Completing the Examination

- Look for pretibial myxedema – non-pitting, skin changes over shins in hypothyroidism.
- With arms folded stand up. Assessing for proximal myopathy, a feature of hypothyroidism.
- With patient stood up, ask them to place a knee on the chair, and test their ankle reflexes one at a time. Hyper-reflexia in hyperthyroidism, and hypo-reflexia in hypothyroidism.
- Thank the patient and wash your hands

1.3 INVESTIGATIONS

1.3.1 PURE TONE AUDIOGRAM

Background

- An audiogram is a graph of frequency (Hz) plotted against intensity (dBHL).
- A Pure Tone Audiogram (PTA) is the main behavioural hearing test for adults and children (>4years old).
    - The thresholds of hearing for a range of tones (250Hz - 8000Hz) are deduced for each ear by the patient responding to the each tone that is heard (threshold is defined as the softest intensity detected 50% of the time).
    - Air and bone conduction thresholds enable initial differentiation between conductive, mixed and sensorineural hearing loss
    - The normal range is -10 to +20 dBHL
- Any asymmetry needs investigating with 'masking' so that the function of each cochlea can be determined.
    - Masking is needed whenever the non-test ear, rather than the test ear could detect the signal presented to the test ear.

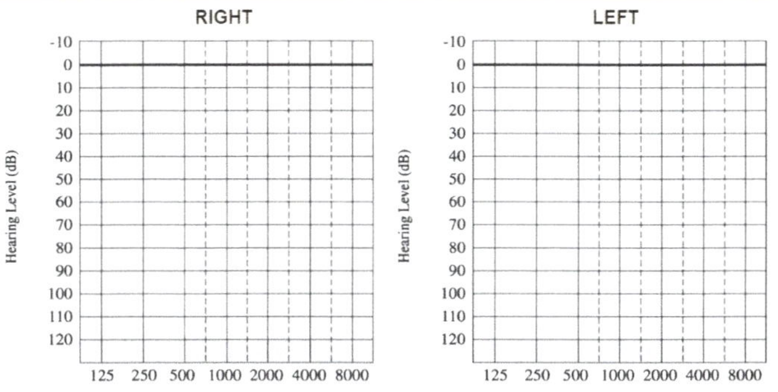

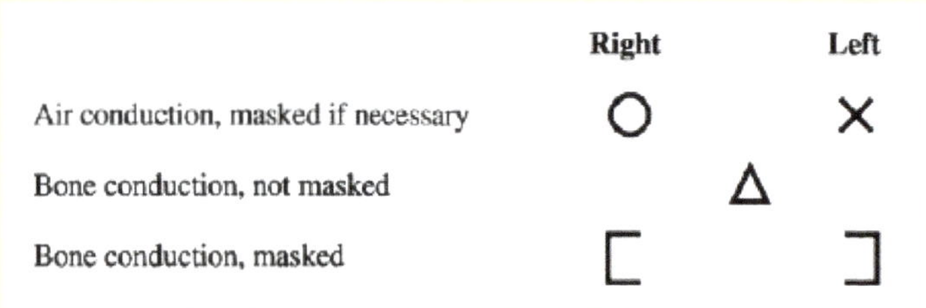

Figure 1.3.1a: Blank template example of an audiogram. The symbols used in clinical audiology in the UK

Interpretation	
Figure 1.3.1b: Conductive Hearing Loss	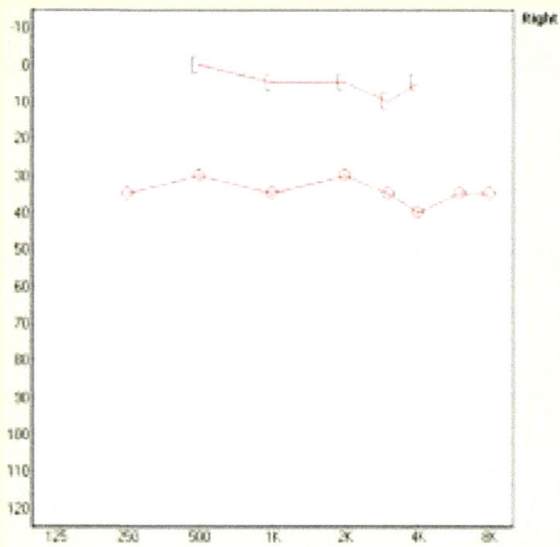

Figure 1.3.1c: Sensorineural Hearing Loss

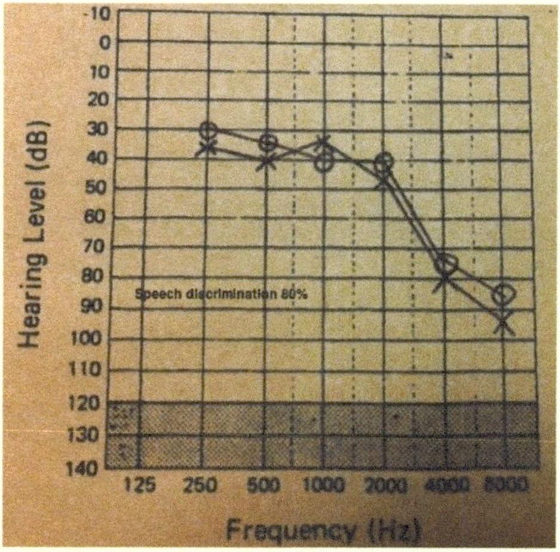

Figure 1.3.1d: Otosclerosis

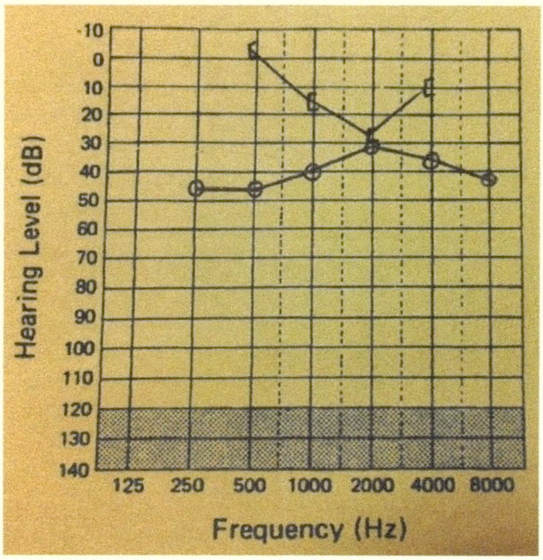

Figure 1.3.1e: Noise-induced Hearing Loss

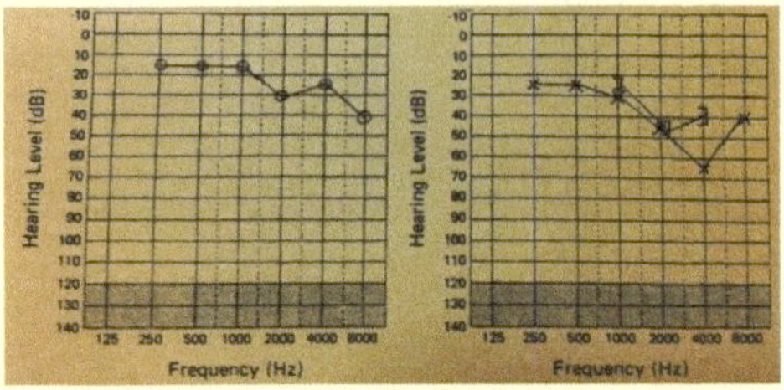

Figure 1.3.1f: Degrees of Hearing Loss

Average threshold dB	Hearing loss
0 - 20	None (normal)
20 - 40	Mild
40 - 70	Moderate
70 - 90	Severe
> 90	Profound

1.3.2 TYMPANOGRAM

Background

- Tympanograms are graphs showing acoustic admittance/impedance as a function of the ear canal pressure (which can be varied from positive to negative)
- Acoustic *admittance* is the amount of sound transmitted through the middle ear system. Acoustic *impedance* is the reciprocal of this (the amount of sound not transmitted/or is reflected back from the tympanic membrane)
- 3 key variables are measured during tympanometry:
    - Ear canal volume (normally 1-1.5ml)
    - Peak acoustic admittance
    - Middle ear pressure
- Hence, tympanometry is an indirect measure of the middle ear status
- The tympanogram will show a peak when the pressure of the middle ear is equal to the pressure in the canal

Interpretation

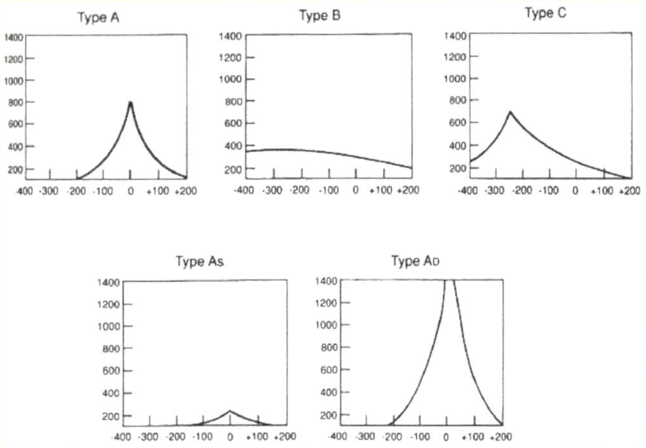

Figure 1.3.2 ***Types of Tympanograms***: Type A -Normal Tympanogram, Type B Flat Tympanogram indicative of OME or perforated tympanic membrane, Type C - Suggests eustachian tube dysfunction due to negative peak, Type As tympanogram indicates possible otosclerosis (A shallow), Type Ad indicates dislocation of ossicles or flaccid TM

1.3.3 RADIOLOGY: CT and MRI

Background

Interpreting radiological investigations such as CT scans and MRI scans can be difficult. Here are a few basic points to help you understand these radiological investigations:

- **Basic key information pertaining to MRI and CT:**
  - Terms: low or high **signals/attenuation** (with CT use the term hypo- or hyper- **dense**). Low signal is black and high signal is white
  - T2 weighted scans means that Water appears White (WW) i.e. high signal
  - T1 weighted scans means that Water appears Black, i.e. Low signal
  - Fat is high signal on both T1 and T2
  - Contrast (gadolinium) is only given in T1; contrast may be seen in blood vessels or in choroid plexus.
  - Normally scans are done as: T2 then T1 then T1 with contrast
  - Very black areas: Bone, Air, Flowing blood (flow voids)

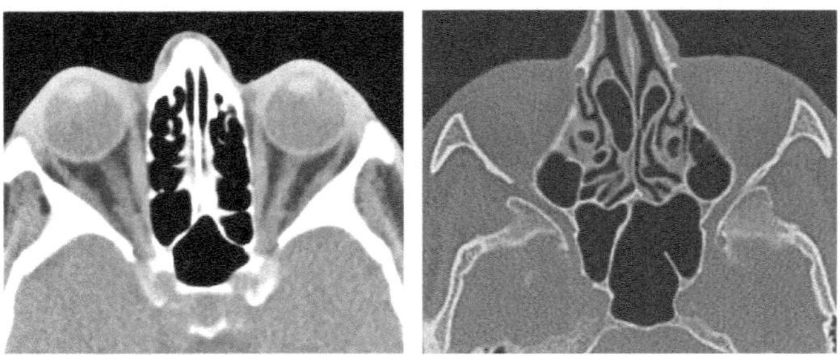

Figure 1.3.3a. Axial CT images throught the nose and paranasal sinuses (soft tissue window and bony window)

Interpretation and Presentation

When looking at a MRI consider the following plan: **'PWCAP'**

- **P**lane
    - Axial
    - Coronal
    - Sagittal
    - Oblique
- **W**indow (for CT scans e.g. soft tissue or bone)
- **C**ontrast given?
    - If yes, then this must be a T1-weighted scan
- **A**natomical location
    - Describe what anatomical sites the scan is focusing on
- **P**athology demonstrated
    - Describe any pathology
    - High or low signal?
    - Which side is the lesion?
    - What are the effects of this lesion? E.g. distortion of other structures?
    - What are the possible differentials?

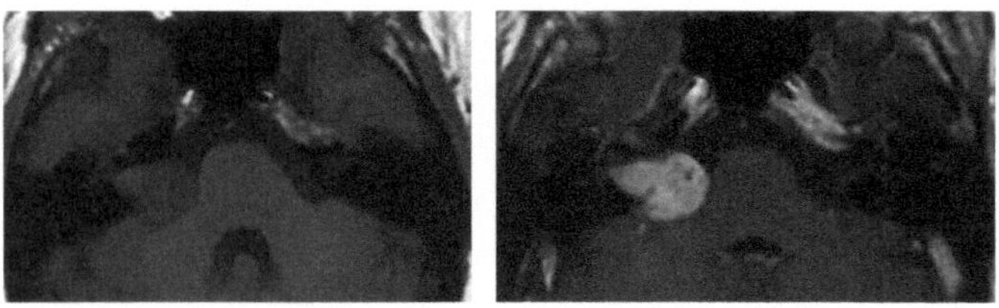

Figure 1.3.3b. Axial MR images taken through the cerebellar pontine angle showing an acoustic neuroma on the right side (1st image is T1 without contrast and the 2nd image is T1 with contrast)

Chapter 2

Ear

2.1 OUTER EAR

2.1.1 EXTERNAL EAR TRAUMA

Clinical scenario

An 8-year-old boy presents with a laceration to his ear following an alleged fall. He has no signs of associated head trauma or other injuries. He has no significant past medical history and is otherwise fit and well. Closer examination of his ear reveals the following injury, which required a few stitches under general anaesthesia.

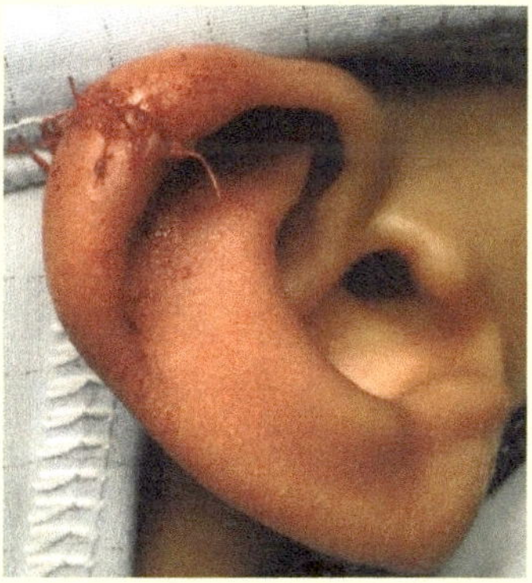

Figure 2.1.1a Pinna laceration

Focusing question	Answer
How would you describe the injury?	• There appears to be a through and through laceration on the superior aspect of the helix of the pinna • There is no significant loss of tissue and therefore primary closure of the wound was possible
Management	**Answer**
What are the main issues relevant in the history?	• Mechanism of injury to determine if it is a clean or dirty wound • Time of injury • Loss of consciousness/ vomiting/ severe headache may indicate serious head injury • Hearing loss suggests middle/inner ear trauma • Clear/bloody discharge from ear/nose suggesting base of skull fracture • Exclude associated injuries (ENT/Non-ENT)

What would be your approach to examine this patient?	• In general, trauma patients should be immediately resuscitated using the primary survey ABCDE approach as per ATLS guidelines
	• Rule out associated head/brain injury
	• Inspection:
	    o Inspect for severity of injury – is it involving the skin/cartilage, length of laceration
	    o Is the wound clean or dirty –

	check for foreign bodies within the wound o Otoscopy - Examine the middle ear for canal trauma/ haemotympanum/ TM perforation that could indicate more severe base of skull or ossicle/inner ear injury o Examine behind the ear for Battle's sign suggesting base of skull fracture o Check facial nerve – may be affected if associated temporal bone fracture o Nystagmus
If there was an associated hearing loss, what investigations would you request?	• Tympanograms • Audiogram – conductive loss suggesting middle ear injury or sensorineural loss suggesting inner ear trauma
What treatments may be required?	• Medical o ABC resuscitation o Anti-Tetanus Booster (IM injection) o Irrigate wound with sterile saline o Antibiotics if contaminated wound

<table>
<tr><td></td><td>• Surgical
    o Surgical closure of the laceration under local or general anaesthetic</td></tr>
<tr><td>Is follow up needed?</td><td>• Yes to check that the wound has healed up satisfactorily and to remove any non-absorbable suture.
• Repeat audiological assessments if hearing loss is noted</td></tr>
<tr><th>Additional Question (s)</th><th>Answer</th></tr>
<tr><td>Draw and label a normal pinna.</td><td>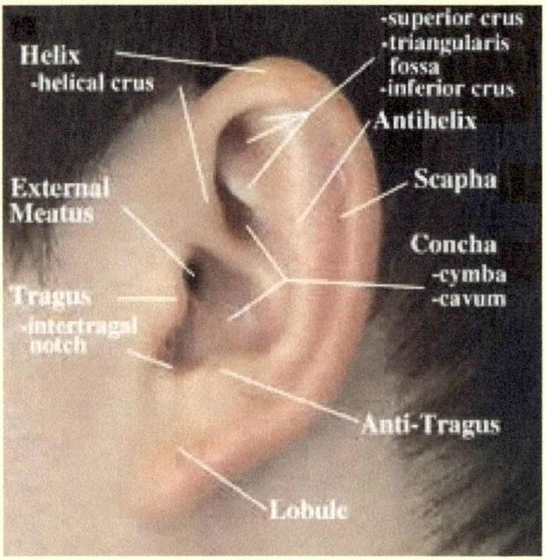
</td></tr>
<tr><td>What is the main function of the pinna?</td><td>• Sound localisation. The shape of the pinna structures aids this.</td></tr>
</table>

2.1.2 PINNA HAEMATOMA

Clinical scenario

A 27-year-old rugby player presents with a swollen, blue-red pinna, following a lateral blow to the ear during a rugby match. He is on no medication and is fit otherwise.

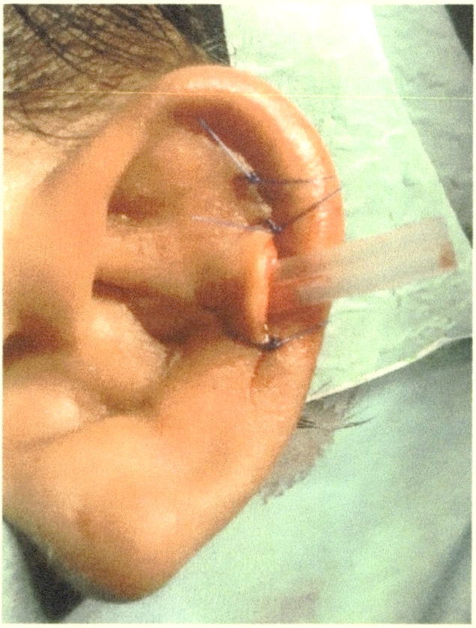

Figure 2.1.2 Incision and drainage of a pinna haematoma. *(Image from ENT Tzar Urgent Care in Otolaryngology)*

Focusing question	Answer
What is the diagnosis?	• Pinna Haematoma
Management	**Answer**
What questions would you ask in this patient?	• Methods of trauma • Time since trauma • Rule out serious head injury: hearing loss, ear discharge, nasal discharge
How would you examine this patient?	• Inspect and palpate haematoma for site, size and lacerations • Examine for any temporal bone or basal skull fractures • Otoscopy for any transmitted injuries from the blow e.g. perforated tympanic membrane
How would you treat this patient?	• Clean and dress any lacerations • Refer for surgical evacuation via incision and drainage of haematoma • Monitor for re-accumulation of haematoma
What complication would you be aiming to prevent?	• 'Cauliflower ear' which results in permanent pinna deformity

Additional Question (s)	Answer
How does pinna haematoma result in 'cauliflower ear'?	• The pinna is made from cartilage which is avascular • The cartilage is supplied with nutrients via its perichondrium covering • A haematoma often forms between the perichondrium and the cartilage resulting in obstruction of nutrient supply • The main complication of this is avascular necrosis, which causes the deformity

2.1.3 PERICHONDRITIS

Clinical scenario

A 21-year-old girl presents with a 48-hour history of erythema, swelling and tenderness of her left auricle. She had her pinna pierced 4 days earlier. Examination reveals the following:

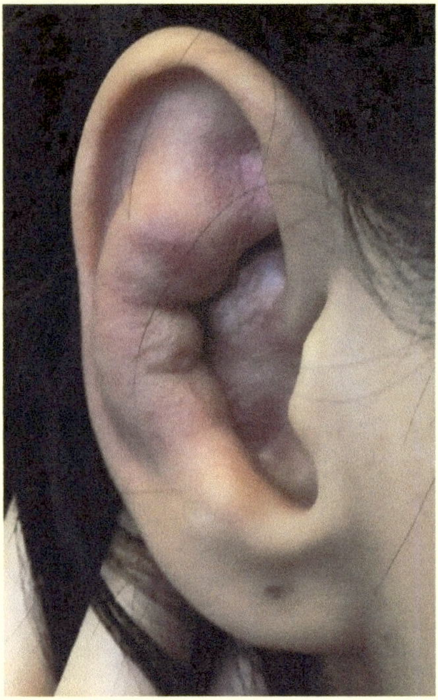

Figure 2.1.3 Inflamed pinna

Focusing question	Answer
What is the most likely diagnosis and the differential diagnosis?	• Perichondritis • Pinna cellulitis • Perichondrial abscess
Management	**Answer**
What questions would you ask in this patient?	• Acute onset of swelling and erythema • Auricular pain • Recent ear trauma/ cartilage piercing • Fever • Recurrent/ relapsing episodes may indicate an underlying autoimmune disease (relapsing polychondritis)

How would you examine this patient?	• Inspection.
	    o Swollen, inflamed auricle. Usually localised.
	    o Area of trauma / piercing
	• Palpation for fluctuant swelling requiring drainage
	• Otoscopy – rule out concurrent otitis externa/media

What possible investigations could you request for this patient?	• Culture any pus. • Bloods for inflammatory markers (FBC/CRP) • Autoimmune screen in relapsing cases

How would you treat this patient?	<ul><li>Remove any piercing</li><li>Medical<ul><li>Oral or IV antibiotics as per hospital microbiology guidelines</li><li>Oral steroids if underlying autoimmune disease</li><li>Analgesia</li></ul></li><li>Surgical:<ul><li>Drain any abscess</li></ul></li></ul>
Additional Question (s)	**Answer**
Define Perichondiritis.	<ul><li>Perichondritis is inflammation of the perichondrium. In the ENT context, it affects the skin and connective tissue surrounding the cartilage of the outer ear.</li><li>Relapsing perichondritis is an autoimmune condition (the ear lobule is normally not affected)</li></ul>
What common microorganism may be responsible for infective perichondritis?	<ul><li>*Pseudomonas aeruginosa*</li></ul>

2.1.4 OTITIS EXTERNA

Clinical scenario
An eighteen-year-old girl presents with a one-week history of an itchy, painful right ear. It is associated with creamy discharge and reduced hearing on that side. She is a keen swimmer who is otherwise fit and well. Otoscopic examination reveals the following:

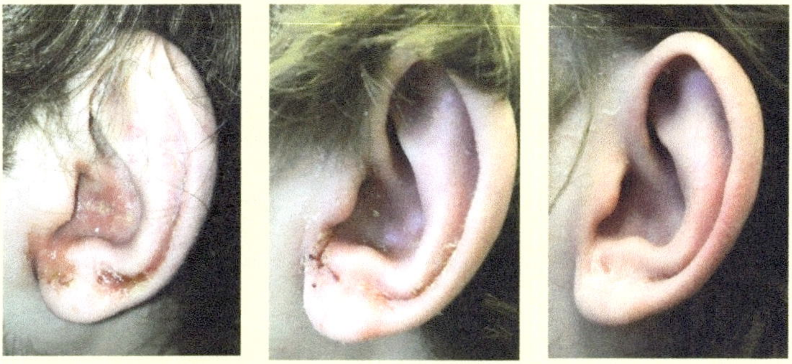

Figures 2.1.4 Otitis externa before and after treatment with antibiotic eardrops and topical steroid ointment.

Focusing question	Answer
What is the most likely diagnosis?	• Otitis Externa: The external auditory canal shows classic features of otitis externa – inflammation, narrowing, debris, creamy coloured discharge.
Management	**Answer**
What questions would you ask in this patient?	• Risk factors: Use of cotton buds, swimming habits – use of ear plugs, hearing aid, atopy/eczema

	• Symptoms:
	  o Otalgia
	  o Hearing loss
	  o Discharge
	  o Pruritus
	• Risk factors for malignant otitis externa: diabetes, immunocompromised/steroids, alcohol excess.

How would you examine this patient?	• Inspection.
	  o Oedema occluding canal, erythema, granulation tissue, discharge, aural polyp
	  o Pinna involvement
	• Assess cranial nerves (in particular facial nerve).
	• Infection localised to the outer hair bearing part of the canal may represent furunculosis.

What possible investigations could you request for this patient?	• Micro-otoscopy to confirm diagnosis; assess canal patency and presence of drum perforation. • Swab for MC&S for bacteria +/- fungi

How would you treat this patient?	• Regular microsuction (aural toilet) • Topical antibiotic drops • Steroid ointments with antibiotics • Advise patient to keep ear dry • If canal is narrowed insert popewick to aid delivery of eardrops • Topical antifungal for otomycosis • Systemic antibiotics if pinna/facial cellulitis • Analgesia
What is your follow up plan?	• Remove popewick after 72 hours • Another follow up appointment 1 week later to confirm improvement.
Additional Question (s)	**Answer**
What organisms are commonly associated with otitis externa?	• Bacterial: *Pseudomonas aeruginosa, Staph aureus, Proteus* • Fungal: *Aspergilus niger, Aspergillus fumigatus, Candida albicans* • Viral: Herpes simplex, Herpes zoster
What other factors predispose to developing Otitis Externa?	• Inflammatory: Eczema, psoriasis, dermatitis • Environmental: Bathing, swimming, heat, humidity, hearing aid use • Trauma: Cotton buds, nails • Inherited: Narrow ear canals

2.1.5 FOREIGN BODY IN THE EAR

Clinical scenario

A 4-year-old child presents to you with his mother, who states that the child has not been responding to his name, and has recently been pulling at his ear. She remembers the child recently playing with small toys.

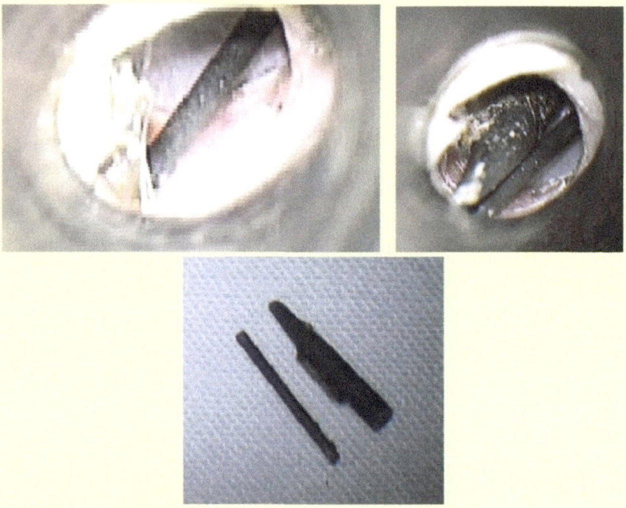

Figures 2.1.5 Foreign bodies (pencil lead) in the left and right ear canals of a child.
(Image from ENT Tzar Urgent Care in Otolaryngology)

Focusing question	Answer
What is the most likely diagnosis?	• Likely foreign body in the external auditory canal
Management	**Answer**
What questions would you ask in this patient?	• Time of, and duration since the event/symptoms • Was the event witnessed? • The possible nature of the foreign body (organic or non-organic?) • Symptoms secondary to foreign body e.g. hearing loss, bloody discharge, otalgia
How would you examine this patient?	• Make the child comfortable and gain their trust • Perform otoscopy examination of both ears to identify any foreign body • Check for traumatic perforations, secondary infections or local damage from the foreign body
What investigation could be done to test the child's hearing? What is it likely to show?	• Pure tone audiogram (young children may require more specialist hearing tests) • Conductive hearing loss secondary to foreign body

What are the treatment options for this patient?	• Keep the patient calm and gain both theirs and parents trust • Using good technique, a trained individual should remove the foreign body e.g. via suction, wax hooks or forceps. This may be done in outpatient setting, or may have to be done under general anaesthesia (which carries its own risks)
Additional Question (s)	**Answer**
How can the external canal be divided anatomically?	• The external canal is divided into two sections and is of sigmoidal shape • The lateral 1/3 is cartilaginous • The medial 2/3 is osseous
What type of substances would you be most worried about as a foreign body in the ear?	• Substances that can corrode are particularly dangerous and warrant urgent removal by professionals e.g. button batteries • Organic matter should also be removed relatively urgently. This may swell and cause pain. They may predispose to infection.

2.2 MIDDLE EAR

2.2.1 PERFORATION OF TYMPANIC MEMBRANE

Clinical scenario

32-year-old male complains of hearing loss and recent onset of tinnitus. He states that these symptoms occurred soon after a recent scuba diving holiday. You suspect a likely perforation of his left tympanic membrane

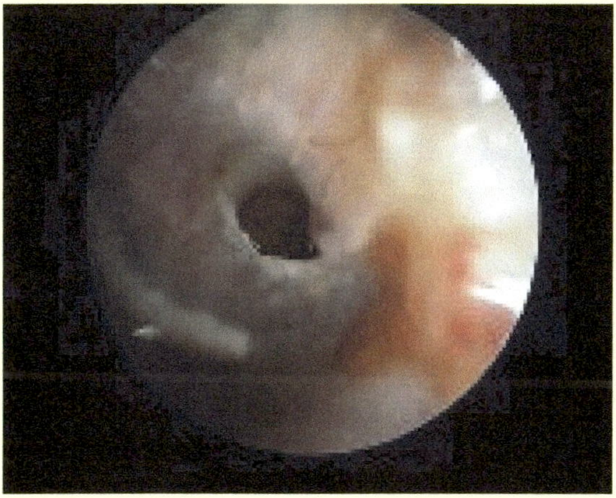

Figure 2.2.1 Traumatic tympanic membrane perforation, classically small, jagged edges, occasionally triangular shaped.

Focusing question	Answer
What are the other causes of tympanic membrane perforation?	• Trauma e.g. blow to the head • Blast injuries • Air travel • Iatrogenic e.g. following otological procedures (syringing of ear) • Non-accidental injury • Secondary to acute otitis media
Management	**Answer**
What signs on examination could you look for in a patient?	• General examination: look for signs of trauma, bruising etc. that may indicate the aetiology • External ear: pinna trauma, blood in canal, chronic ear discharge • On otoscopy: perforation of tympanic membrane
What would Tuning Fork tests show in this patient?	• This would indicate a likely conductive hearing loss • Weber's test would lateralise to the left ear • Rinne's test will be negative on left side (bone conduction>air conduction)
What are the treatment options for this patient?	• Consider audiological assessment • Precautionary management: avoid swimming and avoid water entering ears during bathing using local protocol methods • Discuss with senior if querying non-accidental injury

Additional Question (s)	Answer
What are the two anatomical parts of the tympanic membrane?	• Pars tensa (inferior part of membrane). Larger. • Pars flaccida (superior part of membrane). Much smaller. • Both consist of 3 layers: mucosa, collagen fibres and epithelial but in the pars flaccida the fibrous layer is random and not as organised as in the pars tensa

2.2.2 TEMPORAL BONE FRACTURE

Clinical scenario

A 38-year-old bouncer was brought to hospital after allegedly receiving a blow across the left side of the head with a metal bar; he briefly lost consciousness and now complains of reduced hearing on that side. He is brought to hospital and undergoes a CT scan. The images are shown below.

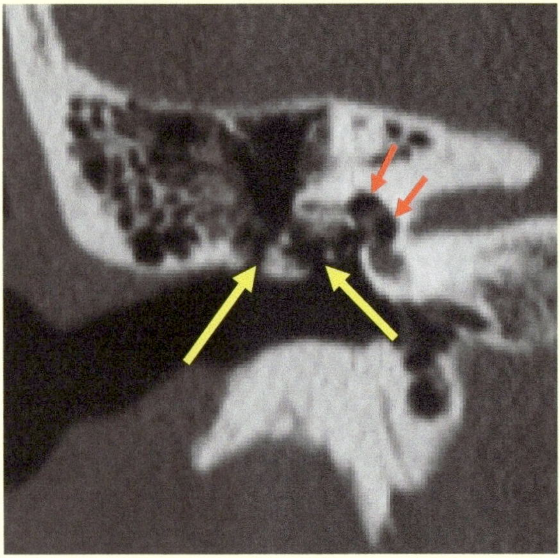

Figure 2.2.2 Coronal CT image showing fractures (yellow arrows) of the temporal bone as well as a pneumolabyrinth (red arrows). *(Image from ENT Tzar Urgent Care in Otolaryngology)*

Focusing question	Answer
What is the most likely diagnosis and the differential diagnosis?	• Longitudinal Temporal bone fracture (80%) (lateral blow to the head) • Transverse temporal bone fracture (Anterior/Posterior blow to the head) • Mixed fracture
Management	**Answer**
What questions would you ask in this patient?	• Mechanism of injury • Vertigo • Hearing loss • Watery discharge from ear/nose (CSF) • Bloody discharge from ear • Facial nerve palsy (immediate or delayed) • Other associated injuries • Head/brain injury
How would you examine this patient? And what is your immediate management?	• Examination 1. Otoscopy – haemotympanum/swelling /EAC laceration/ TM perforation/ serosanguinous discharge/ clear discharge 2. Battle's sign, Peri-orbital echymoses 3. Nystagmus 4. Full cranial nerve examination 5. Test each of the 5 branches of VII nerve. Grade weakness according to House-Brackmann classification 6. Signs of raised ICP 7. Full neurological examination

What possible investigations could you request for this patient?	• Bloods. FBC/coagulation/group+save/ crossmatch • Radiology – High resolution CT temporal bone, CT head/brain • Special tests. Pure tone audiogram, Tuning fork tests • Beta-2 transferrin test to confirm CSF otorrhoea/rhinorrhoea
How would you treat this patient? Think about the individual possible problems.	• Immediate management 1. Acute stabilisation of patient using ATLS primary and secondary survey • External ear canal laceration, haemotympanum or ruptured TM: 1. Conservative, avoid straining. • Nystagmus and nausea/vomiting: 1. PRN prochloperazine (Stemetil) 2. Vestibular rehabilitation exercises. 3. Usually resolves completely after 3-6months • Facial nerve palsy: 1. Immediate complete palsy: exploration/decompression/repair of facial nerve 2. Immediate incomplete: suggests a functional non-severed nerve, recovers with time. 3. Delayed palsy –10 days oral steroid if not contraindicated

	• CSF leak: • Conservative: **1.** Bed rest, head elevation and stool softeners **2.** No sneezing, no coughing, no straining, no nose blowing **3.** Usually closes by 1 week • Medical: Prophylactic antibiotics, risk of meningitis is approximately 15% (*haemophilus and streptococcus*) • Surgical: If leak persists: referral to neuro-otologist for surgical closure. Consider lumbar drain • Hearing loss: • Medical: ▪ Contra-lateral routing of sound (CROS) aid or Bone conduction hearing aid (BCHA) for single sided deafness. • Surgical ▪ Tympanoplasty or ossiculoplasty for conductive hearing loss (surgical exploration after 2 months if hearing loss is <30dB, unless only hearing ear).

What would be your follow up plan	• Repeat audiogram after 8 weeks • Water precautions until outpatient follow-up
Additional Question (s)	**Answer**
What is the difference in fracture pattern between the two main fracture types?	• **Longitudinal fractures** are longitudinal to the long axis of the petrous portion of the temporal bone. Runs through the middle ear and ear canal leading to conductive hearing loss and haematorrohea. It may involve carotid canal. Haemotympanum and ruptured TM can occur. Facial nerve involvement uncommon. • **Transverse fractures** run perpendicular to the long axis of the petrous temporal bone and are more likely to run through the otic capsule and cause CSF leak, facial palsy and total nerve hearing loss (dead ear occurs) associated with severe vertigo and nystagmus to opposite ear. Haemotympanum can occur but TM perforation less common.

2.2.3 FACIAL NERVE PALSY

Clinical scenario

A 75-year-old man presented with inability to move the right side of his face and a painful right ear. He had no significant past medical history and was generally fit and well. He was not taking any medications and was not allergic to any known medicines. His wife recently passed away. Examination revealed some vesicles in the conchal bowl of his right ear.

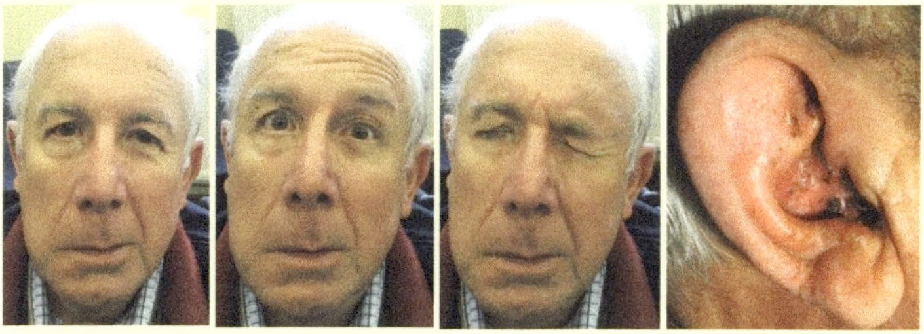

Figure 2.2.3a Clinical photographs showing right sided facial nerve weakness and pinna of patient.

Focusing question	Answer
What is the most likely diagnosis and the differential diagnoses?	• **Ramsay Hunt Syndrome:** The presence of a facial nerve palsy associated with vesicles in the distribution of a sensory branch of the facial nerve are classical features of Ramsey hunt syndrome, which is thought to be due to the dormant herpes virus that resurfaces during a stressful life situation (e.g. bereavement).

	• **Bell's Palsy:** Idiopathic facial nerve palsy (this is a diagnosis made when all other causes are excluded)
Management	**Answer**
What questions would you ask in this patient?	• Acute onset of unilateral facial weakness • Facial pain- may suggest parotid pathology • Ear pain- may suggest middle ear pathology • Neurological symptoms suggest upper motor neuron pathology such as a stroke • Exclude serious head injury • Exclude iatrogenic cause – i.e. recent otological surgery • History of recent travel to forested areas where Lyme's disease is present e.g. Sweden, Canada and England • Enquire about stressful situation which may affect the immune system
How would you examine this patient?	• Inspection. o Most importantly identify whether weakness in UMN or LMN: in LMN the forehead in **NOT** spared. If there is forehead sparing seek urgent medical input due to possible stroke o Test each of the 5 branches of VII nerve. Grade weakness according to House-Brackmann

	classification • Palpation. Parotid lumps. • Otoscopy – cholesteatoma, haemotympanum, herpes zoster vesicles in EAC, malignant otitis externa • Special tests. Check lacrimation, taste and salivation
What possible investigations could you request for this patient?	• Bloods. Blood tests for sarcoidosis (ACE) and Lyme's disease (serology) • Radiology. A CT scan is necessary before the diagnosis of Bell's palsy could be made • Special tests. Pure tone audiogram and stapedial reflexes

How would you treat this patient?	• Supportive: Eye care: glasses for eye protection, eye pad to close eye lid at night, artificial tears
	• Medical:
	  o Bell's Palsy/Ramsay-Hunt: oral prednisolone – reducing dose starting 60mg OD and oral antiviral – 800mg five times/day
	  o Acute otitis media/mastoiditis – IV antibiotics and steroids

What would be your follow up plan?	• Repeat audiogram after 8 weeks • Water precautions until outpatient follow-up • If suspected Bell's palsy/Ramsay Hunt syndrome, patient can be discharged and

	reviewed in one week to monitor progress • Advise that recovery is usually within a few weeks but can take 12 months • Up to 20% may have incomplete recovery
Additional Question (s)	**Answer**
Describe the anatomy of the facial nerve	• The facial nerve has a very complex tortuous course which may be divided into various segments: (i) intracranial, (ii) intratemporal and (iii) extracranial • Intracranial segment begins from the facial nerve nucleus and travels with CNVIII into the internal auditory meatus of the temporal bone • Intratemporal segment within the temporal bone (labyrinthine and tympanic parts) travels horizontally, and then takes a 90 degrees turn posteriorly where it gives off the greater petrosal nerve. It then turns 90 degrees inferiorly and gives off the nerve to stapedius and chorda tympani. • The extracranial segment begins at the stylomastoid foramen. It gives off a branch to the posterior belly of digastric and another branch to stylohyoid. The facial nerve travels between the deep and superficial lobes of the parotid gland. Within the gland, it divides into the 5 terminal branches: temporal,

	zygomatic, buccal, marginal mandibular and cervical.
What the different functions of the facial nerve?	• The facial nerve has 4 functions: motor, general sensory, parasympathetic and special sensory • Motor to muscles of facial expression, stapedius muscle, posterior auricular muscle and buccinators • General sensory to conchal bowl of ear • Parasympathetic to lacrimal submandibular and sublingual glands • Special sensory i.e. taste to anterior 2/3 of tongue
What are the other causes of facial nerve palsy?	• ***Congenital*** (e.g. mobius syndrome involving multiple cranial nerve palsies) • ***Acquired***: trauma (e.g. temporal bone fracture), infection (e.g. herpes virus), inflammation (e.g. sarcoidosis) and neoplasia (e.g. adenoid cystic carcinoma of parotid gland). In the case of Ramsay Hunt syndrome, vesicles may be present in the distribution of one or more of the non-motor branches of the facial nerve e.g. conchal bowl or chorda tympani. • When no specific cause for the facial nerve palsy is found after thorough investigations, the diagnosis is known as Bell's palsy (hence this is a diagnosis of exclusion)

Describe one grading system for facial nerve palsy.	• ***House-Brackman*** grading system where grade 1 is normal and grade 6 is no movement whatsoever; grade 3 is complete eye closure and grade 4 is incomplete eye closure 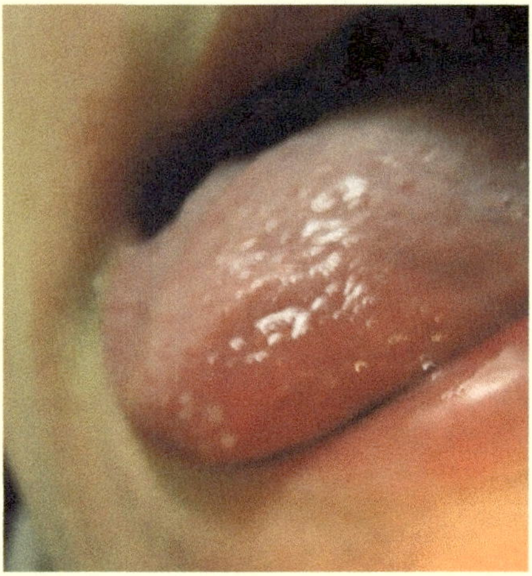 **Figure 2.2.3b.** Clinical photograph showing herpes vesicles in the distribution of chorda tympani of another patient.

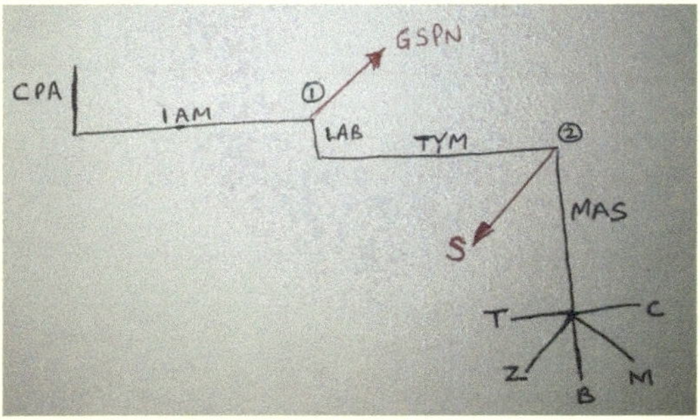

Figure 2.2.3c. Schematic diagram showing the segmental anatomy of the facial nerve with its 5 terminal branches. CPA cerebellar pontine angle, IAM internal auditory meatus, LAB labyrinthine, TYM tympanic, MAS mastoid, T temporal, Z zygomatic, B buccal, M mandibular, C cervical, 1 first genu and 2 second genu, GSPN greater superficial petrosal nerve, S stapedial nerve.

2.2.4 ACUTE OTITIS MEDIA

Clinical scenario
A 10-year-old child presents with a 3-day history of increasing left sided otalgia following an upper respiratory tract infection. He has spiked a fever in the past 24 hours. The child has no significant past medical history. Otoscopic examination reveals the following:

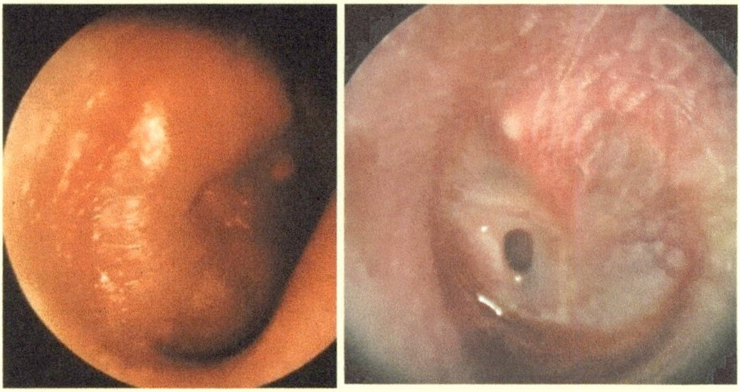

Figure 2.2.4 Bulging tympanic membrane consistent with acute otitis media and ruptured tympanic membrane in AOM. *(Image from ENT Tzar Urgent Care in Otolaryngology)*

Focusing question	Answer
Describe the findings	• Red inflamed bulging tympanic membrane • The appearance is dull with a loss of the light reflex • This is in keeping with acute otitis media

What organisms are commonly associated with acute otitis media?	• Bacterial: *Streptococcus pneumonia, Haemophilus influenza, Moraxella catarrhalis* • Viral – may precede bacterial infection
Management	**Answer**
What questions would you ask in this patient?	• Preceding URTI • Otalgia • Reduced hearing in affected ear • Tinnitus in affected ear • Fevers • Discharge – following tympanic membrane perforation • Immunosuppression - Consider immune deficiency in recurrent cases or unusual pathogens • Exclude complications- facial weakness, headache, photophobia, neck stiffness.
How would you examine this patient?	• Inspect for mastoid swelling / post-auricular fluctuance (to rule out mastoiditis) • Otoscopic examination of tympanic membrane – inflamed +/- perforation • Check facial nerve function • Inspect for signs of meningism / extracranial complications

<table>
<tr><td>What possible investigations could you request for this patient?</td><td><ul><li>Bloods for inflammatory markers</li><li>Swab any discharge for MC&S</li></ul></td></tr>
<tr><td>How would you treat this patient?</td><td><ul><li>Supportive: analgesia and antipyretics first 72 hours</li><li>Medical:<ul><li>Oral antibiotics after 72 hours for 2 weeks as per local microbiology guidelines</li><li>Topical antibiotics if concurrent otitis externa</li></ul></li><li>Surgical: Myringotomy if associated complications such as facial nerve palsy.</li></ul></td></tr>
<tr><td>Additional Question (s)</td><td>Answer</td></tr>
<tr><td>What are the associated complications with this disease?</td><td><ul><li>Temporal – acute mastoiditis, acute petrositis, Gradenigo's syndrome (ASOM, ipsilateral abducent nerve palsy, pain in distribution of ipsilateral trigeminal nerve)</li><li>Extracranial - LMN facial nerve palsy, Citelli's abscess (spread to digastric fossa), Bezold's abscess (spread to sternocleidomastoid), Labyrinthitis</li><li>Intracranial – meningitis, extradural/subdural/intracranial abscess, lateral sinus thrombosis</li></ul></td></tr>
</table>

	• **Other** – Tympanic membrane perforation producing mucopurulent discharge
What are the long-term sequelae of acute otitis media?	• Non-suppurative middle ear effusion • Sensorineural hearing loss • Tympanic membrane perforation • Tympanosclerosis • Ossicular chain erosion

2.2.5 ACUTE MASTOIDITIS

Clinical scenario
A 5-year-old child complains of left sided ear pain. You notice the child's left pinna is protruding, and is no longer symmetrical when compared to the right ear. You suspect acute mastoiditis. On further questioning, the mother tells you her daughter recently complained of ear pain, and fever.

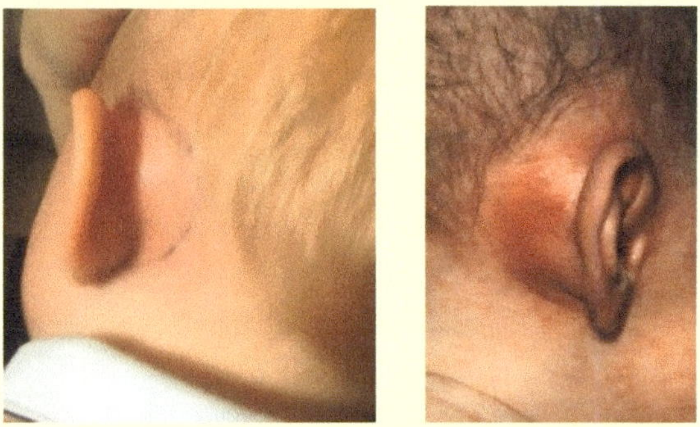

Figures 2.2.5 Early and late acute mastoiditis. *(Image from ENT Tzar Urgent Care in Otolaryngology)*

Focusing question	Answer
What illness is likely to have preceded the acute mastoiditis?	• Acute otitis media

Management	Answer
What questions would you ask in this patient?	• Preceding illnesses and symptoms • Systemic upset e.g. fever • Pain posterior to ear • Intracranial symptoms e.g. drowsiness, nausea and vomiting, headache • Past medical history e.g. immunosuppression? • Previous surgical history e.g. mastoidectomy
What would you look for on examination?	• Protrusion of ear on affected side due to mastoid abscess • Post auricular region will have a fluctuant and boggy swelling • Post auricular tenderness on palpation • Otoscopy may show acute otitis media • Examine neurology further for other intracranial complications e.g. meningitis, raised intracranial pressure, cranial nerve palsies (facial nerve)
How would you investigate this patient?	• Bloods: inflammatory markers, FBC, blood cultures, pre-op workup • Imaging: CT temporal bone may be useful, but diagnosis is usually clinical. MRI scanning can help to detect other intracranial complications

How would you treat this patient?	<ul><li>Stabilise and admit patient</li><li>Senior review urgently</li><li>IV to oral Antibiotics as per hospital protocol</li><li>Surgery may be required e.g. mastoidectomy</li></ul>
Additional Question (s)	**Answer**
What are the anterior and posterior borders of the middle ear?	<ul><li>Anterior border is the Eustachian tube</li><li>Mastoid antrum forms the posterior border. This is one reason why acute otitis media can result in acute mastoiditis, as it provides a route for infection to spread.</li></ul>

2.2.6 EUSTACHIAN TUBE DYSFUNCTION

Clinical scenario

A 24-year-old woman presents complaining of a sensation of "blocked ears" bilaterally with reduced hearing following a recent URTI. She has a childhood history of glue ear.

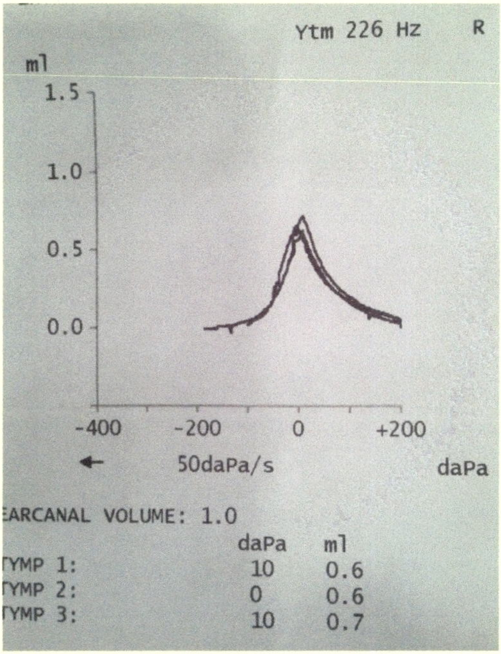

Figure 2.2.6a Tympanographs showing Eustachian tube dysfunction (ie no separation of the graphs before, during and after swallowing).

Focusing question	Answer
What are the common causes of Eustachian tube dysfunction?	• Narrow Eustachian tube (infants) • Rhinosinusitis/sinusitis • Nasopharyngeal tumours • Ciliary dysfunction

Management	Answer
What questions would you ask in this patient?	• Symptoms: Epistaxis, unilateral symptoms (may suggest nasopharyngeal tumour), hearing loss • Risk factors: URTI, sinus disease, congenital ciliary disorders, smoking (can cause ciliary dysfunction)
How would you examine this patient?	• Inspection – dull grey TM if middle ear effusion • Examine Fossa of Rosenmuller on FNE for nasopharyngeal tumour
What possible investigations could you request for this patient?	• Pure tone audiogram • FNE – nasopharyngeal tumour/sinus disease • CT sinuses for surgical planning if surgery is being considered.
How would you treat this	• Medical: steroid nasal spray, hearing aid

patient?	<ul><li>Surgical: myringotomy +/- grommet if associated effusion, functional endoscopic sinus surgery</li><li>Malignancy: - CT/MRI for staging, Biopsy for histological diagnosis, MDT discussion and appropriate management</li></ul>
Additional Question (s)	**Answer**
Describe the anatomy of the Eustachian tube.	<ul><li>The Eustachian tube is 3-4cm in length and extends from the middle ear to the lateral wall of nasopharynx posterior to the inferior turbinate</li><li>Divided into two segments: lateral one third is the bony; medial two thirds is fibrocartilaginous. The Eustachian tube is narrowest where these two portions meet.</li><li>The tube is lined with respiratory type (pseudostratified ciliated columnar) epithelium.</li></ul>
What is the function of the Eustachian Tube?	<ul><li>Drainage of middle ear secretions into the nasopharynx</li><li>Protection of middle ear from nasopharyngeal secretions and sound pressures</li><li>Pressure regulation of the middle ear</li></ul>

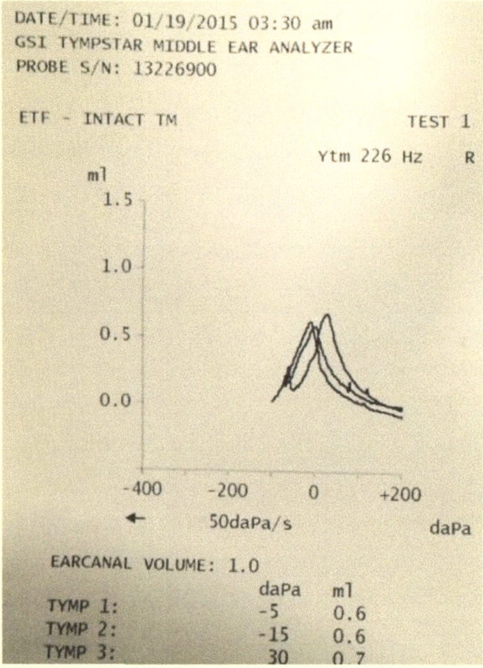

Figure 2.2.6b Separation of the tympanographs before, during and after swallowing is indicative of normal Eustachian tube function

2.2.7 OTITIS MEDIA WITH EFFUSION

Clinical scenario

A five-year-old child presents with hearing loss. His parents are concerned that he has difficulty hearing the teacher and that his speech development is behind other children. He has no other medical problems and there is no family history of medical problems. All other developmental milestones are being achieved appropriately.

Examination reveals the following:

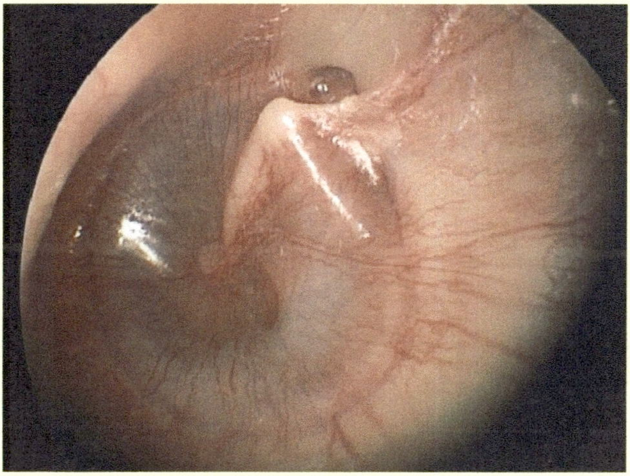

Fig 2.2.7: Otitis Media with middle ear effusion (note the dull tympanic membrane and increase vascularity)

Focusing question	Answer
Describe the findings	• Dull grey bulging tympanic membrane in keeping with otitis media with middle ear effusion (Glue ear)

Management	Answer
What questions would you ask in this patient?	• Persistent or intermittent hearing loss • Learning difficulties and speech delay • Behavioural problems • Recurrent infections • Global developmental delay / congenital diseases e.g. Down's Syndrome
How would you examine this patient?	• Otoscopy - Tympanic membrane inspection dull red/grey/yellow drum. Bulging or retracted. Air bubbles or fluid level may be visible. • Inspect for dysmorphic features
What possible investigations could you request for this patient?	• Pure tone audiometry – Conductive hearing loss • Tympanogram – flat trace
How would you treat this patient?	• Conservative o Watch and wait for spontaneous resolution. Reassure parents. Review in 3 months with repeat hearing

	test. • Surgical ○ Grommet insertion +/- adenoidectomy if conservative management ineffective
What is your follow up plan?	• Review 3 months after grommet insertion and repeat hearing test to monitor symptoms
Additional Question (s)	**Answer**
Describe how middle ear effusion develops	• Eustachian tube dysfunction leads to chronic reduction in middle ear pressure. This causes an inflammatory response and production of thick mucus fluid "glue".
What are the sequelae of glue ear?	• Acute infection causing acute otitis media • Tympanic membrane retraction pocket which may lead to cholesteatoma

2.2.8 CHOLESTEATOMA

Clinical scenario

A 25-year-old woman presents with a 2-month history of increasingly foul smelling right ear discharge. She has a past history of middle ear infections but is otherwise fit and well. Following microsuction the otoscopic examination reveals the following:

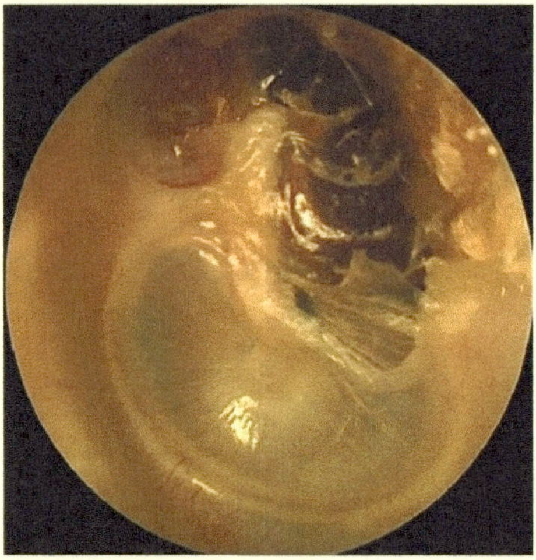

Figure 2.2.8: Otoscopic photograph of left tympanic membrane with attic cholesteatoma

Focusing question	Answer
What is the most likely diagnosis	• Acquired Cholesteatoma

Managemen t	Answer
What questions would you ask this patient?	• Onset and duration- discharge lasting for weeks should prompt you to think about cholesteatoma! • Foul creamy discharge • Complications: hearing loss both conductive and/or sensorineural (if invades inner ear), vertigo, meningitis symptoms, facial weakness.
What would you look for on examination ?	• Inspection – Microsuction of discharge to allow proper inspection. • Check for attic crust – must be removed • Tympanic membrane perforation • Tympanic membrane retraction pocket • Polyp • Granulation tissue
What possible investigation s could you request for this patient?	• Micro-otoscopy • Pure tone audiometry • CT scan to investigate the extent of disease and pre-operative planning

How would you treat this patient?	• Conservative (if patient not suitable for operative intervention)
	  o Interval scanning to check disease progression
	  o Regular aural toilet
	• Medical

	<ul><li style="list-style-type:circle">Topical antibiotics for associated otitis externa</li><li style="list-style-type:circle">Oral antibiotics for acute otitis media</li></ul><ul><li>Surgical<ul><li>Mastoidectomy and disease resection + tympanoplasty</li></ul></li><li>Follow Up<ul><li>Regular follow up to check for disease recurrence</li></ul></li></ul>
Additional Question (s)	**Answer**
What factors predispose to developing cholesteatoma?	<ul><li>Congenital – usually manifests in the first year of life as a result of persistent epidermoid ectoderm</li><li>Acquired – factors causing disruption to the normal migration of the epithelium of the tympanic membrane<ul><li>Eustachian tube dysfunction</li><li>Recurrent middle ear effusion</li><li>Tympanic membrane operations</li><li>Tympanic membrane perforation</li></ul></li></ul>
What are the histopathological findings in this disease?	<ul><li>Macroscopic<ul><li>Pearly white mass</li><li>Associated friable polyp or granulation</li></ul></li><li>Microscopic<ul><li>Benign keratinizing squamous cell epithelia</li></ul></li></ul>

What are the potential complication s associated with this condition?	Cholesteatoma enlarge and become locally invasive, replacing the middle ear mucosa and resorbing bone. Complications are similar to otitis externa:
	
	• Extracranial
	  o Otitis externa
	  o Ossicular erosion
	  o Lower motor neurone facial nerve palsy
	• Intracranial
	  o Meningitis
	  o Extradural/subdural/intracerebr al abscess

2.2.9 PRESBYACUSIS

Clinical scenario

A 75-year-old gentleman presents with progressive hearing loss, which is worse in the presence of background noise and he is finding it increasingly difficult to socialise. He suffers from hypertension but is otherwise well and active. She has no history of excessive noise exposure and examination is normal. Audiogram reveals the following:

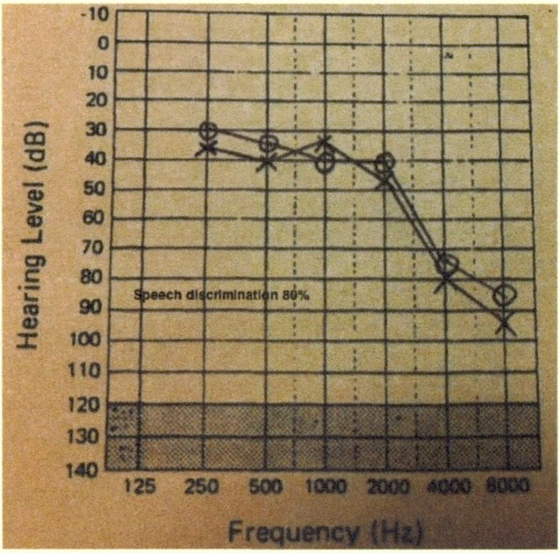

Figure 2.2.9 PTA of the patient showing air conduction thresholds in both ears

(Image from ENT Tzar DOHNS and MRCS(ENT) OSCE Guide)

Focusing question	Answer
What type of hearing loss does this audiogram show? How would you describe the changes?	• Bilateral sensorineural hearing loss • Sloping high frequency loss • (These findings are suggestive of presbyacusis)
What is the aetiology of this condition?	• Progressive age-related deterioration affecting peripheral and central auditory pathways
Management	**Answer**
What questions would you ask in this patient?	• Onset • Affect on daily living • History noise exposure • Bilateral or unilateral hearing loss • Tinnitus/vertigo
How would you examine this patient?	• Inspection – examination is usually normal
What possible investigations could you request for this patient?	• Pure tone audiogram • MRI of internal acoustic meatus if unilateral symptoms (to exclude acoustic neuroma)
How would you treat this patient?	• Supportive: Hearing aids, Home aids and adaptive devices e.g. induction coils in the telephone/television

What would be your follow up?	• Audiology services to follow-up and support hearing aid user
Additional Question (s)	**Answer**
Name some of the possible causes of conductive and sensorineural hearing loss?	Conductive • Foreign body • Wax • Acute otitis media ± effusion • Tympanic membrane perforation or scarring • Otosclerosis Sensorineural • Noise-induced • Presbyacusis • Vestibular schwannoma • Meniere's disease • Drug-induced • Inflammatory • Infective • Genetic

2.2.10 NOISE-INDUCED HEARING LOSS

Clinical scenario

A fifty-year-old gamekeeper presents with progressive hearing loss worse on the right side, he complains of difficulty listening to conversations in the presence of background noise. He is otherwise fit and well. Otoscopic examination is normal. Pure tone audiograms reveal the following:

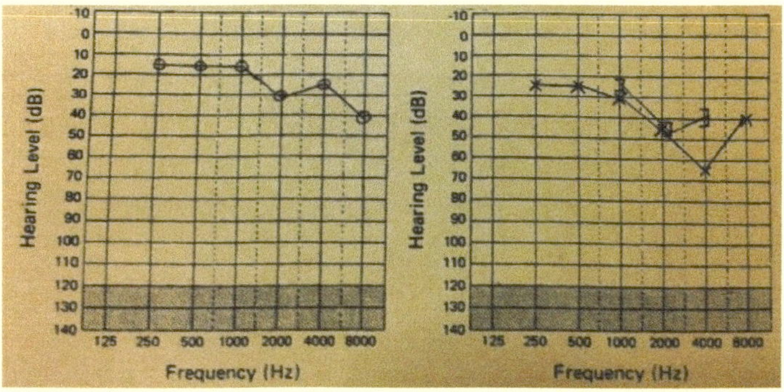

Figure 2.2.10 Insert photo of audiogram showing noise induced hearing loss

Focusing question	Answer
What is the diagnosis?	• Noise induced hearing loss – audiograms will show a typical dip at 4-6 kHz
Management	**Answer**
What questions would you ask in this patient?	• Onset • Duration • Occupation

	• Thorough history of noise exposure and whether ear protection used o In this example ask which is the dominant hand (as the side of use is most likely to be affected) • Family history (to rule out hereditary causes)
How would you examine this patient?	• Otoscopic examination – will usually be normal
What possible investigations could you request for this patient?	• Pure tone audiogram – sensorineural loss
How would you treat this patient?	• Supportive: hearing protection, avoid further noise exposure, referral to hearing therapist, education on hearing hazards • Medical: Hearing aid
What would be your follow up?	• Medico-legal advice for compensation may be required if secondary to occupational exposure.

Additional Question (s)	Answer
What is the aetiology of this disease?	• Repeated excessive noise exposure causes progressive damage to the rows of outer hair cells then the inner hair cells. Damage typically occurs at >90dB
What is the aetiology in this case? What explains the right-sided loss?	• Regular use of a shotgun as a gamekeeper causes noise induced hearing loss. • Right-handed shooter – the right ear is closer to the barrel of the gun.

2.2.11 OTOSCLEROSIS

Clinical scenario
A 30-year-old woman presents with progressive hearing loss in the right ear following a normal pregnancy. She remembers that her mother suffered from similar symptoms at her age that necessitated an operation. She is otherwise fit and well. Examination is normal. Pure tone audiogram shows the following:

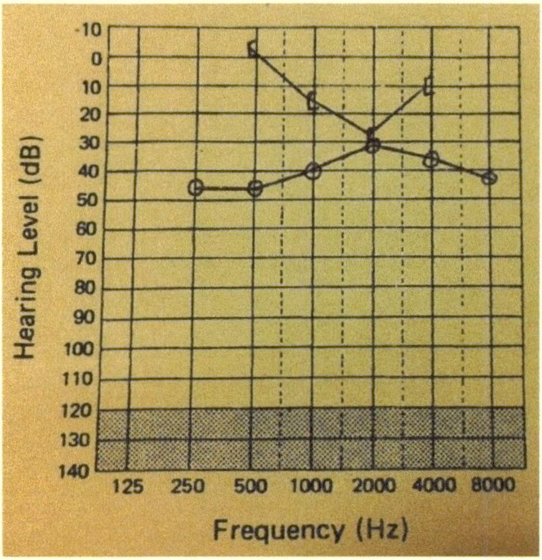

Fig 2.2.11: Pure Tone Audiogram of patient

Focusing question	Answer
What is the diagnosis?	• Otosclerosis – presence of Carhart's notch (dip at 2000Hz) on pure tone audiogram

What is the differential diagnosis?	• Ossicular discontinuity • Fibro-osseous foot plate fixation • Paget's disease • Congenital foot plate fixation • Congenital cholesteatoma • Osteogenesis imperfecta
Management	**Answer**
What questions would you ask in this patient?	• Hearing loss – sometimes better in noisy surroundings • Onset in women commonly associated with pregnancy, menstruation and menopause • Tinnitus • Vertigo
How would you examine this patient?	• Inspection. – Otoscopy is usually normal. 10% have a pink tinge to TM from dilated blood vessels (Schwartze's sign).
What possible investigations could you request for this patient?	• Pure tone audiogram – Typically conductive hearing loss at low frequencies. Sensorineural loss with cochlear involvement • Speech audiometry • CT scan if cochlear involvement suspected
How would you treat this patient?	• Supportive: Hearing aid • Surgical: Stapedectomy

Additional Question (s)	Answer
What is the genetic aetiology? What is pathogenesis of this disease?	• Autosomal dominant condition • NB there may be a linked measle viral infection • Lamellar bone is replaced by woven bone • Affects bone of the otic capsule only (endochondrial layer) causing fixation of stapedial footplate. Otospongiosis may also affect other parts such as the round window and cochlea.

2.3 INNER EAR

2.3.1 BENIGN PAROXYSMAL POSITIONAL VERTIGO (BPPV)

Clinical scenario

A 28-year-old man presents with intermittent episodes of vertigo exacerbated when turning her head particularly to the left and when turning. The intermittent vertigo followed a 48 period of severe unsteadiness associated with vomiting (labyrinthitis). The episodic vertigo last less than one minute. There is no associated tinnitus or hearing loss. He is otherwise fit and well and not on any regular medications.

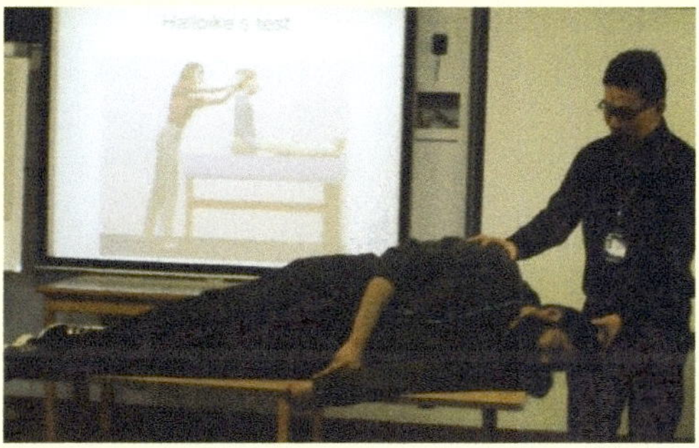

Figure 2.3.1a. Transient vertigo induced by turning to the left side

Focusing question	Answer
What is the most likely diagnosis?	• Benign Paroxysmal Positional Vertigo (BPPV)

What are differential diagnoses for intermittent vertigo?	• Peripheral (vestibular) causes: Meniere's disease, acute vestibular failure • Central causes: cerebrovascular disease, migraine, malignancy, multiple sclerosis • Iatrogenic: ototoxic drugs (diuretic, antibiotics e.g. aminoglycosides) • Other: cervical neck disease, cerebellopontine angle tumour (unilateral symptoms), cholesteatoma, syphilis

Management	Answer
What questions would you ask in this patient?	• Onset, frequency, duration. • Triggers - head turning is a classical trigger. • Associated symptoms – vomiting, (tinnitus may suggest Meniere's disease). • Past medical history. • Drug history (especially ototoxic drugs) • Head trauma
How would you examine this patient?	• Full otological and neurological examination, nystagmus • Romberg's and Unterberger's test. Unterberger's test is a test to lateralise vestibular pathology. The patient is asked to march on the spot, with arms out in front. A turning of >45 degrees after 50 steps indicates a positive test. The direction of turning points to the side of pathology. • Dix-Hallpike test.

What possible investigations could you request for this patient?	• Audiogram • MRI/CT if suspicion of central cause/ cerebellopontine angle tumour • Cervical spine x-ray
Describe the Dix-Hallpike test	• Seat patient on examination couch with eyes open. Reassure patient. • Turn head to 45 degrees to the affected side extending the neck. Support head between your hands. • Lay patient down with head extended 30 degrees over end of the couch. Ask patient if this provokes symptoms and observe for the presence of nystagmus for 30 seconds. • Return patient to upright position and repeat with head turned to opposite side.
What findings would you expect to find in BPPV?	• Onset of rotatory nystagmus after 5 seconds. Fast down beating saccades towards the affected ear. Nystagmus lasts 10-20 seconds and is fatigable on repetition. Symptoms of vertigo are provoked. • Immediate onset of nystagmus that persists suggests central cause.

What is the treatment for this patient?	Supportive: • Vestibular rehabilitation – reassurance, counselling, Brandt-Daroff exercises (a series of exercises that patients perform and progressively relieve symptoms by displacing otoliths) • Epley manoeuvre to reposition displaced otoliths Medical: • Prochlorperazine, betahistine Surgical: • Posterior semicircular canal obliteration
Describe Epley's Manoeuvre	• Sit patient on examination couch. Turn head 45 degrees towards the affected side • Lay patient down with head supported between your hands, extended 30 degrees over the end of the couch for 30 seconds. • Turn head 45 degrees to the contralateral side • Roll patient onto the contralateral side lying on their side with affected ear facing upwards, and head facing 45 degrees downwards • Sit patient up with head turned away from affected side • Return head to normal position. • Repeat Hallpike test following the manoeuvre. If nystagmus still present repeat Epley's manoeuvre.

What is your follow up plan?	• Follow-up in 1 week following the Epley manoeuvre. • Symptoms can recur and may require repeat manoeuvre. 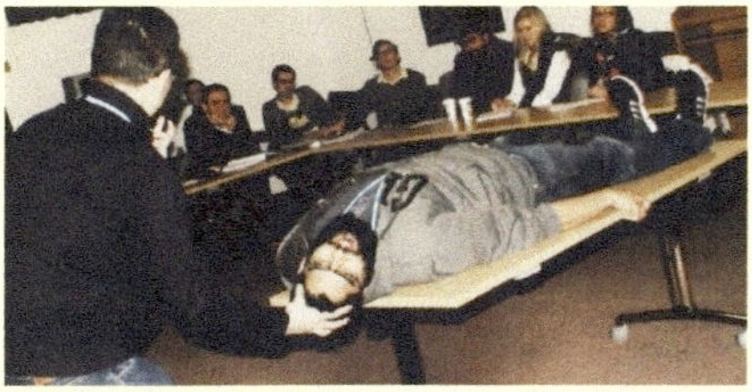 **Figure 2.3.1b** Epley manoeuvre in action
Additional Question (s)	**Answer**
What is the underlying aetiology of BPPV?	• Otoliths (calcium crystals) are displaced from their normal position within the utricle into the semi-circular canal. Upon head movement there is abnormal movement of endolymph in the semi-circular canal due to the presence of the otolith debris resulting in vertigo.
Describe the anatomy of the vestibular system	• 3 semi-circular canals orientated perpendicularly – each canal consists of the crura dilating to form the ampulla containing the crista ampullaris and cupula. The semi-circular canal contains endolymph. These sense angular acceleration. • 2 otolith organs – utricle and saccule containing hair cells covered by an otolithic membrane. These sense linear acceleration.

2.3.2 MENIERE'S DISEASE

Clinical scenario

A 42-year-old gentleman presents with a history of debilitating episodes sensation of the "room-spinning" lasting 2-3 hours. These episodes are associated with nausea, ringing in ears, hearing loss and feeling of fullness particularly in the right ear. They have been occurring in increasing frequency but between episodes he is symptom free. Examination in clinic is normal. Audiogram shows the following:

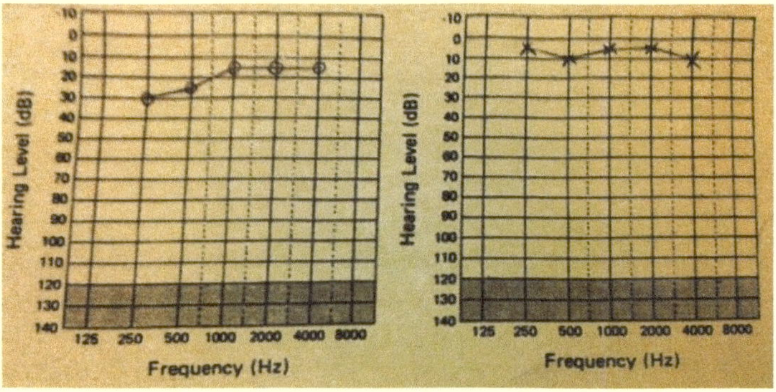

Figure 2.3.2 Meniere's syndrome of the right ear.
(Image from ENT Tzar DOHNS and MRCS(ENT) OSCE Guide)

Focusing question	Answer
What is the most likely diagnosis?	• Meniere's disease

What are other causes of intermittent vertigo?	• Peripheral Vestibular causes: BPPV, acute vestibular failure • Central causes: Cerebrovascular disease, migraine, malignancy, multiple sclerosis • Iatrogenic: ototoxic drugs (diuretic, antibiotics e.g. aminoglycosides) • Other: Cervical neck disease, Cerebellopontine angle tumour (unilateral symptoms), cholesteatoma, syphilis
Management	**Answer**
What questions would you ask in this patient?	• Carefully define what they mean by “dizziness”. This is not synonymous with vertigo. • Duration- hours is more suggestive of Meniere’s disease whereas days duration is more likely labyrinthitis or vestibular neuritis. • Frequency, onset, triggers, nature of symptoms, head trauma: Relapsing and remitting episodes of vertigo lasting 1-24 hours +/- hearing loss/tinnitus/fullness/nausea/vomiting • Drug history- ototoxic drugs? • Past medical history- past neurological problems? Cardiovascular risk factors- predispose to posterior circulation TIA.

How would you examine this patient?	• Full otological and neurological examination • During episodes: - nystagmus, normal otoscopy, exacerbation with movement Between episodes: - normal examination • Hallpike test – (see BPPV) • Romberg's and Unterberger's tests • General cardiovascular examination
What possible investigations could you request for this patient?	• Audiogram – fluctuating low frequency sensorineural loss • MRI if cerebellopontine angle tumour suspected (unilateral signs and symptoms) • Vestibular function tests if unclear.
How would you treat this patient?	• Supportive: Change in diet (e.g. reduce caffeine, salt), symptom diary • Medical: Betahistine and prochlorperazine – during attacks • Surgical: Grommet insertion, Cortical mastoidectomy with endolymphatic sac decompression, labyrinthectomy, vestibular nerve section, ultrasound destruction of vestibular labyrinth • Long-term symptom support and reassurance

Additional Question (s)	Answer
What is the aetiology of this condition?	• Primary cause unknown: ?labyrinthine ischaemia or ?viral trigger • Subsequent endolymph expansion and increase in endolymphatic pressure affects inner ear structures causing symptoms

2.3.3 LABYRINTHITIS

Clinical scenario
A 30-year-old man presents with sudden onset of severe dizziness with associated nausea and vomiting. The dizziness was preceded by URTI and left sided otalgia. He has no other medical problems and no significant family history. On examination he is unable to move his head due the severity. Eye examination reveals a nystagmus.

Focusing question	Answer
What is the most likely diagnosis and the differential diagnosis?	• Acute labyrinthitis • Labyrinthine fistula • Meningitis • Cerebral abscess
How is labyrinthitis classified?	• Perilabyrinthitis – Labyrinthine fistula following mastoid surgery. • Paralabyrinthitis – vertigo associated with chronic otitis media. Nystagmus occurs towards affected ear • Serous labyrinthitis – bacterial labyrinthitis causing vertigo with subsequent recovery of cochlea and vestibular function • Suppurative labyrinthitis – vertigo with irreversible loss of inner ear function

How is nystagmus graded?	• Grade 1 – nystagmus present when looking in direction of fast component • Grade 2 – nystagmus also present when straight ahead • Grade 3 – nystagmus present when looking straight ahead and in direction of fast and slow component
Management	**Answer**
What questions would you ask in this patient?	• Onset, trigger, duration, frequency, preceding symptoms, associated symptoms, exacerbation with movement • Past medical history • Past mastoid surgery
How would you examine this patient?	• Otoscopy – normal/ features of chronic or acute otitis media • Micro-otoscopy may reveal fistula • Nystagmus – initially grade 3 and improves with compensation • Fistula sign • Full neurological examination – meningitis/ cerebral abscess • Romberg's test • Unterberger's test • Head Impulse test = test for peripheral vestibular pathology. Positive test is when the eyes make no response or a corrective saccade

	to rapid turning of the head in the direction of the pathology.
What possible investigations could you request for this patient?	• Bloods – inflammatory markers • Audiogram • CT head – meningitis/abscess • Ear swab any discharge for MC&S
How would you treat this patient?	• Supportive: Bed rest • Medical: IV fluids, anti-emetic, vestibular sedative (prochlorperazine), antibiotics if infection, Cooksey-Cawthorne exercises (vestibular rehabilitation exercises) • Surgical: Grafting of labyrinthine fistula
What is your follow up plan?	• Monitor recovery of hearing loss and vestibular function • Vestibular rehabilitation exercises • Counselling if delayed compensation/irreversible loss of function

Additional Question (s)	Answer
Describe Romberg's test	• Ask patient to stand, feet together eyes closed. Reassure the patient beforehand and be ready to catch them if they lose balance. • Positive test - Patient will fall towards side of peripheral vestibular lesion
Describe Unterberger's test	• Reassure the patient and ask them to march on the spot with the eyes closed and arms held straight out in front • Positive Test = patient rotates more than 30 degrees towards the side of labyrinthine lesion
Describe the Head Impulse test	• Ensure prior to performing this test that the patient does not suffer from cervical spine disease • Examine active and passive neck rotation • Patient to fix gaze at some point behind the examiner • Gently rotate the head 30 degrees from the midline to right and left • Acutely rotate the head back towards the midline and assess whether the gaze lost fixation which led to a re-fixation saccade; this suggests loss of vestibulo-occular reflex on the side the head was turned towards.

	• If fixation was maintained this helps exclude a labyrinthine pathology.

2.3.4 VESTIBULAR SCHWANNOMA

Clinical scenario

A fifty-year-old woman presents with a three-month history of progressive unilateral hearing loss and ringing in her ears. She denies any other symptoms and is otherwise fit and well. There is no family history of hearing loss. Her audiogram revealed a unilateral sensorineural hearing loss. Her MRI scan is shown below.

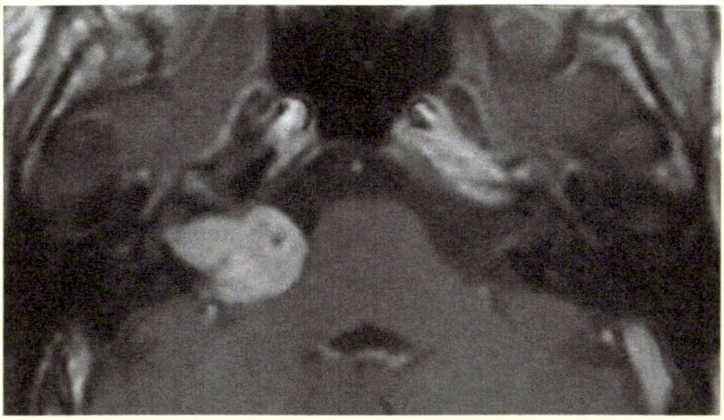

Figure 2.3.4 Axial MR image (T1 weighted with contrast) showing a right cerebellar pontine angle lesion consistent with a vestibular schwannoma)

Focusing question	Answer
What is the most likely diagnosis?	• Vestibular Schwannoma (acoustic neuroma) most commonly arises from superior vestibular nerve.
What are the differential diagnoses?	• Other cerebellopontine angle tumours – meningioma, facial nerve neuroma, cerebellar tumour,

	cholesterol granuloma, aneurysm • Congenital cholesteatoma • Vertebral/basilar artery aneurysm
Management	**Answer**
What questions would you ask in this patient?	• Symptoms can be divided into otological and neurological • Otological: unilateral deafness, unilateral tinnitus, sudden onset hearing loss • Neurological: trigeminal nerve symptoms, ataxia, diplopia (VIth), dysphagia (IXth/Xth), reduced consciousness/coma (terminal) • Past medical history (note: neurofibromatosis type 2 is associated with bilateral acoustic neuromas)
How would you examine this patient?	• Otological phase: - normal otoscopy, hypaesthesia in posterior ear canal (Histelberger sign). • Neurological phase: - Loss of corneal reflex (V), nystagmus, cranial nerve palsies (VI, IX, X)
What possible investigations could you request for this patient?	• Pure tone audiometry • MRI - Internal auditory meatus and cerebellar pontine angle

How would you treat this patient?	<ul><li>Conservative: Annual MRI to monitor expansion e.g. elderly patients</li><li>Surgical: Surgical resection - translabyrinthine approach/ middle fossa route/ Retrosigmoid approach</li><li>Radiological: gamma-knife surgery. Precise targeting by ionising radiation.</li></ul>

2.3.5 CENTRAL CAUSES OF VERTIGO

Clinical scenario
A 75-year-old gentleman presents with 2-day history of unsteady gait and dizziness. He is an ex-smoker with a history of diabetes, ischaemic heart disease and hypertension. Examination reveals an ataxic gait and up/down beating nystagmus.

Focusing question	Answer
What is the most likely diagnosis?	• Cerebrovascular accident, likely to be of the posterior circulation.
What are the other central causes for vertigo?	• Migraine • Intracranial tumour • Multiple sclerosis
Management	**Answer**
What questions would you ask in the history?	• Onset, duration, frequency of vertigo • Previous episodes • Associated symptoms – tinnitus/hearing loss/neurological deficit/headaches/aura • Trauma • Past medical history • Smoking history • Drug history
How would you examine this patient?	• Full neurological examination including cranial nerves • Nystagmus assessment – up/down

	beating • Gait assessment • Unterberger's test • Romberg's test • Dix-Hallpike test – immediate onset of nystagmus and persistent • Full otological examination • Auscultate for carotid bruits
What investigations could you order?	• Bloods – inflammatory markers, HbA1C, glucose • Audiogram • CT head • MRI brain

How would you treat this man?	Depends on underlying diagnosis
	• Medical:
	    o Thrombolysis - ischaemic cerebrovascular event
	    o Analgesia/triptans/ergotamines – migraine
	    o Steroids/interferon therapy – multiple sclerosis
	• Surgical: carotid endarterectomy may be indicated depending on specific cause.

Chapter 3

Nose and Sinuses

3.1 NOSE

3.1.1 NASAL TRAUMA

Clinical scenario

An 28year old student presents to A&E following an alleged assault when walking home. He has had a nosebleed which seems to be resolving but is now complaining of his pain around his nose and a sensation of his nose having changed shape.

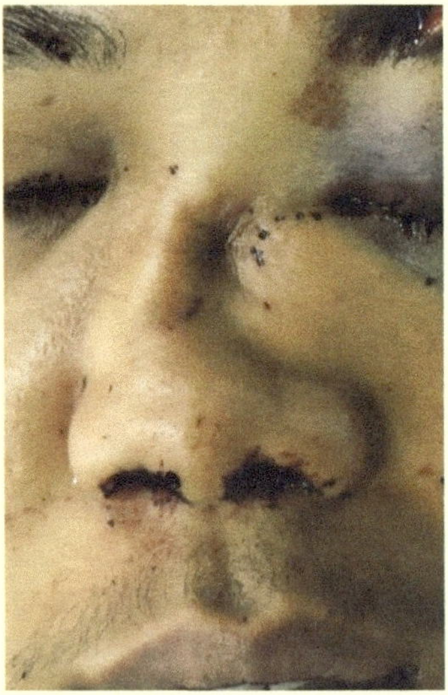

Figure 3.1.1 Clinical photograph showing left nasal deviation due to depressed left nasal bone and upper lateral cartilage.

Focusing question	Answer
What is the most likely diagnosis?	• Nasal fracture.
Management	**Answer**
What would be the first step in your management? What are the salient points in your history?	• Resuscitate according to ATLS guidelines. A broken nose may just be a manifestation of serious head and neck injury. Be aware injury may have occurred elsewhere. • When did this happen? Timing is important- fractures are best reduced within 2 weeks of injury after allowing swelling to settle but before too much callus has developed (see below). • Further details of injury: Low vs. high impact injury, mechanism. • Symptoms of head injury (such as loss of consciousness, amnesia, neurological deficit) or other facial injuries. • Previous nasal injuries or surgery. Important to compare before vs now. Ask how the patient thinks their nose is different, or ask for old photographs. • Past medical history: to include coagulopathies or use of blood thinning medications • Note: people involved in contact sports are more prone to such injuries and advice should be given to them accordingly.

How would you examine this patient? And what is your immediate treatment?	• Inspection.
	    o External nasal deviation, laceration
	    o Signs of base of skull fracture: Battle's sign, Racoon eyes, CSF otorrhoea/rhinorrhoea
	• Full cranial nerve examination including ocular movements, and infraorbital sensation (Vth nerve function)- orbital injury may have occured. Full neurological examination if head injury suspected.
	• Palpation of face. Facial fractures
	• Anterior rhinoscopy: Nasal airway patency, septal haematoma, and rhinorrhoea.
	• Otoscopy: Perforation, otorrhoea, CSF leak, signs of trauma to external auditory canal.

What investigations could you order?	• Usually no investigations are required. • If considerable blood loss order blood tests: FBC, INR, Group and Save. • Radiological investigations not indicated for simple uncomplicated nasal fractures – often carried out for suspected facial fractures

What would be the urgent treatment plan for him?	• If open wound present: irrigate the wound with saline, close using glue/steristrips/suture.
	    o Tetanus vaccination
	    o Prescribe empirical antibiotics (oral sufficient)

#	• If suspected nasal fracture consider Manipulation Under Anaesthesia (MUA)
	    o Can be done immediately in A&E if swelling not excessive.
	    o However patients are usually reviewed at 7 days post-trauma for swelling to improve.
	    o The fracture can be reduced under local or general anaesthesia.
	    o At the latest, MUA should be carried out within 2-3 weeks post-injury. (After this the nasal bones will fix and MUA will be more difficult).

What would you do if patients present after 3 weeks following such injuries?	• For patients who have presented late, septorhinoplasty can be considered. However this is a much larger operation and is not considered in children due to the possibility of affecting growth.
Additional Question (s)	**Answer**

Name some of the bones and cartilages that make up the skeleton of the nose?	• Lateral wall: maxilla, palatine bone, medial pterygoid plate.
	    o 3 turbinates (superior, middle, inferior).
	• Medial wall (nasal septum):
	    o Cartilage: Septal cartilage
	    o Bones: Vomer, perpendicular plate of ethmoid, maxillary bone,

	palatine bone. • Floor: palatine process of maxilla, palatine bone.

Can you name 2 serious complications of nasal fractures?	• Septal haematoma: collection of blood in the cartilage of nasal septum
	  o Requires urgent aspiration or drainage in a controlled environment (usually best in theatre).
	  o Can result in nasal saddle deformity
	• CSF leak/rhinorrhea.
	  o Usually due to fracture of cribriform plate
	  o If suspected, order an urgent CT scan
	  o Many close spontaneously however some require surgery.
	  o Treat with IV Antibiotics due to the potential risk of meningitis

3.1.2 FOREIGN BODY IN THE NOSE

Clinical scenario
You are asked to see a 5-year-old girl who has obvious unilateral foul-smelling discharge. On looking at the child, it is evident that the area around the left nostril looks inflamed and sore with active discharge. The father reports that his daughter was recently seen dismantling a toy.

Focusing question	Answer
What is the most likely diagnosis?	• Nasal foreign body
Management	**Answer**
What questions would you ask in this patient?	• Was there an event that was witnessed? • Does anyone suspect a particular foreign body? • The possible nature of the foreign body (organic or non-organic?) • Symptoms secondary to foreign body e.g. rhinitis or sinusitis symptoms, nasal blockage, snoring, difficulty breathing • Time of, and duration since the event or symptoms • Does the child have a habit of nasal picking/inserting foreign bodies?
How would you examine this patient?	• Make the child comfortable and try to gain the child's trust.

	• Look around the nostril for signs of inflammation indicating vestibulitis (common following foreign body), discharge (unilateral discharge is a foreign body until proven otherwise), halitosis. • Perform anterior rhinoscopy of both nostrils and examine for foreign body.
How would you treat this patient?	• Identify nature and location of the foreign body via examination • Remove using Jobson-Horne probe or Tilley's forceps. • Sometimes, if the child does not cooperate, this will have to be done under general anaesthesia. • N.B: Corrosive materials such as batteries require urgent removal.

3.1.3 EPISTAXIS

Clinical scenario

An 85-year-old lady presented with right-sided epistaxis. She has a history of ischaemic heart disease and has cardiac stents in situ. She lives alone and has poor mobility. Her medications include amlodipine, aspirin and clopidogrel. She has no known drug allergies.

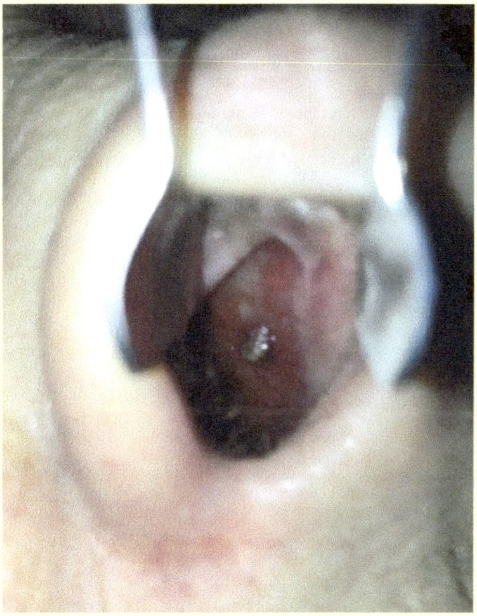

Figure 3.1.3a: Right sided epistaxis caused by a fragile vessel in Little's area

<table>
<tr><th>Focusing question</th><th>Answer</th></tr>
<tr><td>What are the common causes of epistaxis?</td><td><ul><li>Trauma, e.g. nasal injury, nose picking, nasal surgery.</li><li>Systemic disease: Hypertension, coagulopathies</li><li>Blood thinning medications: aspirin, clopidogrel, warfarin</li><li>Neoplastic</li></ul></td></tr>
<tr><th>Management</th><th>Answer</th></tr>
<tr><td>What would you like to do first regarding her management?

What questions would you ask in the history?

How would you</td><td><ul><li>Resuscitate the patient using the ABCDE approach</li><li>Severe epistaxis can compromise the airway as well as circulation.</li></ul><ul><li>How long, how often, how much blood on each occasion (indicates amount and rate of blood loss)</li><li>Side: Unilateral vs. bilateral</li><li>Does it initially start from the front of the nose (anterior epistaxis) or through the mouth (posterior epistaxis)</li><li>Recent history of trauma</li><li>Past medical history</li><li>Family history (e.g. of coagulopathies)</li><li>Medication history (antiplatelets, anticoagulants)</li><li>Weight loss/night sweats (systemic disease)</li></ul></td></tr>
</table>

examine this patient?	<ul><li>Inspection.<ul><li>Anterior rhinoscopy using Thudicum's speculum. Try to identify bleeding point.</li><li>Look inside mouth for blood (may suggest posterior epistaxis).</li><li>Flexible nasendoscopy to look through entire length of nose- may help to identify source of bleeding, especially posterior bleeds.</li></ul></li></ul>
What investigations could you order?	<ul><li>Bloods. FBC, Clotting, Group and Save.</li><li>Radiology not routine. MRI if neoplasia suspected (rarely required).</li></ul>
What would be the urgent treatment plan for her?	<ul><li>Conservative:<ul><li>First aid: lean forward, pinch lateral cartilage of nose together.</li><li>Ice packs (forehead, back of neck)</li></ul></li><li>Medical<ul><li>Resuscitation of patient (IV access, fluids, blood)</li><li>Correct INR, blood pressure</li></ul></li><li>Nasal cauterisation if bleeding point identified<ul><li>Naseptin cream after cauterisation (10 day course) (Avoid if nut allergy)</li></ul></li></ul>

<table>
<tr><td></td><td>

- Nasal packing (anterior or posterior)
  - Anterior: Merocel, Rapid rhino, BIPP
  - Posterior: Foley catheter
- Surgical
  - Ligation of artery – commonly sphenopalatine artery
- Radiological embolisation

</td></tr>
<tr><th>Additional Question (s)</th><th>Answer</th></tr>
<tr><td>Which blood vessels are responsible for epistaxis? Describe the arterial supply to the nose.</td><td>

- Branches of internal carotid artery: anterior and posterior ethmoidal arteries.
- Branches of external carotid artery: greater palatine artery, sphenopalatine artery, superior labial artery.
- Little's area (Kiesselbach's plexus) is most common site of bleeding

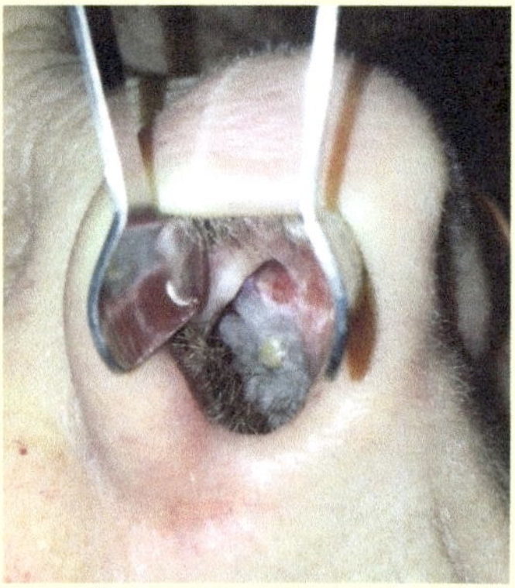

Figure 3.1.3b Cauterised Little's area

</td></tr>
</table>

Other Relevant Clinical Photographs

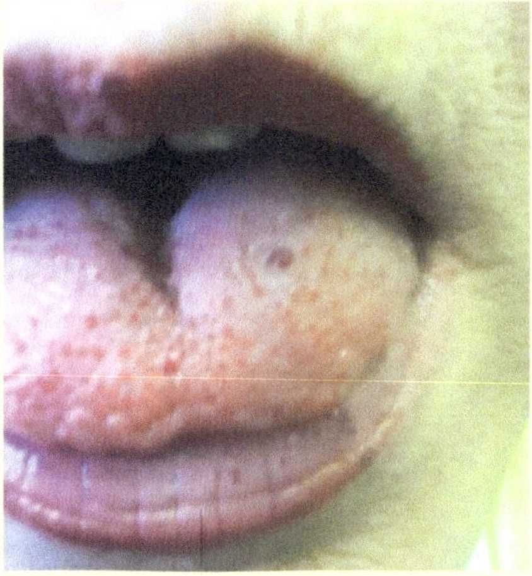

Figure 3.1.3c. Clinical photograph showing telangiectasia on the mucous membranes. Patients with Hereditary Haemorrhagic Telangiectasia (Osler Weber Rendu Syndrome) are prone to significant epistaxis.

3.1.4 SEPTAL PERFORATION and GRANULOMATOUS DISORDERS

Clinical scenario

A 70-year-old man complains of an intermittent whistling sound when breathing. Recently he has had a few nosebleeds and a feeling of a blocked nose.

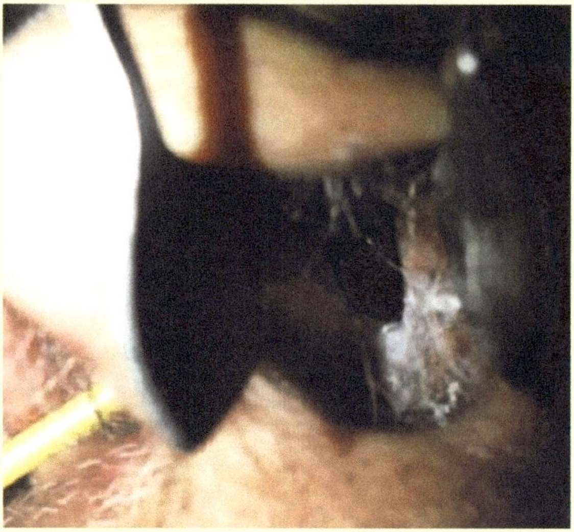

Fig 3.1.4: Anterior Septal Perforation

Focusing question	Answer
What is the most likely diagnosis?	• Septal perforation

Management	Answer

What questions would you ask in the history and how would you examine the patient?	• Symptoms: whistling, epistaxis, nasal crusting, nasal obstruction. Foul smell may emanate from the nasal crust.
	• Consider systemic disease that may cause septal perforation. This includes vasculitis, and cocaine usage.
	• Ask about previous nasal injury or surgery.
	• Inspection.
	    o Anterior rhinoscopy
	    o Flexible nasendoscopy

What investigations would you request?	• Bloods: FBC, U&Es, ESR, ANCA, ACE, syphilis tests (TPA/VDRL)
	• Urinalysis
	• Radiology
	    o CXR/CT Chest
	    o CT sinuses (bony destruction)
	• Biopsy for histology

How would you manage this patient?	• Conservative: majority do not require any intervention.
	• Medical
	    o Saline douche
	• Surgical
	    o Silastic septal button
	    o Surgical repair of perforation

Additional Question (s)	Answer

Give some causes of septal perforation?	• Granulomatous disease
	  o Autoimmune: Wegener's, polyarteritis nodosa, SLE
	  o Chronic infection: TB, syphilis
	  o Sarcoidosis
	• Trauma: nose picking
	• Drugs: cocaine
	• Neoplastic

How do treatment options differ for those with granulomatous disease?	• Medical therapy is preferred: Long-term steroids, immunosuppression • Septal button is preferred over other forms of surgery because outcome is poor especially with large perforations

3.1.5 NASAL POLYPS

Clinical scenario

A 35-year-old lady with a history of asthma presents with a long-standing blocked nose and persistent nasal discharge from both sides of her nose. She is on regular inhalers and frequently requires steroids for her asthma. On examination of her nose, you see obvious polyps in both sides of the nose.

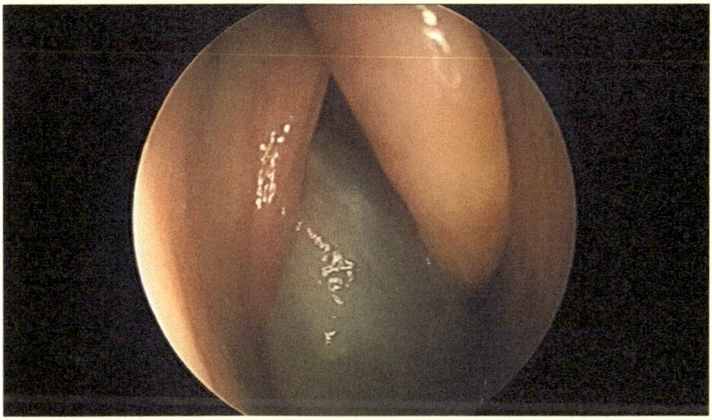

Figure 3.1.5. A large nasal polyp in the middle meatus (between the lateral nasal wall and the middle turbinate)

Focusing question	Answer
Name some of the causes of nasal polyps?	• Allergy • Rare hereditary conditions: Cystic fibrosis, Kartagener's Syndrome
Management	**Answer**
What common symptoms would you ask this patient?	• Nasal blockage - dominant • Nasal discharge • Smell/taste disturbance • Ask about red flag symptoms associated with head and neck cancer. Nasopharyngeal cancer is one of your differential diagnoses.
How would you examine this patient?	• Anterior rhinoscopy • Flexible/rigid nasendoscopy to visualise entire length of nose.
How would you differentiate a nasal polyp from the inferior turbinate?	• Polyps are grey in colour, turbinates are pink • Polyps are insensitive to touch, turbinates are sensitive
How would you investigate this patient?	• Allergy testing: Skin-prick or RAST • Blood tests to detect systemic disease: e.g. ACE, ANCA levels. • Radiology - CT scan to detect sinusitis (often associated with polyps) or malignancy if suspected • Biopsy for histology (if malignancy

	suspected)

How would you treat this patient?	• Conservative:
	  o Allergen avoidance
	• Medical
	  o Steroids (note: steroids have systemic side effects)
	    - Sprays (lowest dose hence are safest)
	    - Drops (avoid use for over 6 weeks due to systemic side effects)
	    - Oral steroids (only if severe, short course)
	  o Antihistamines
	• Surgical: Functional endoscopic sinus surgery (FESS) + polypectomy

Additional Question (s)	**Answer**
What is an antrochoanal polyp and how does it present?	• Unilateral sinonasal polyp, often presents in young men • Usually originates in maxillary sinus and extends through ostium into nasal cavity, and beyond through the choana. It may be visible upon oral exam in the posterior pharynx. • Often larger than normal polyps – can present with unilateral nasal obstruction

How would you investigate it?	• Radiological (CT or MRI) • Biopsy for histology
What is the treatment?	• Surgical removal (FESS + polypectomy).- surgery is preferred mode of treatment. • Steroids (topical or oral) can give temporary relief of symptoms
What is Samter's triad?	• A triad of nasal polyps, asthma and aspirin intolerance

3.1.6 RHINITIS

Clinical scenario

A 35-year-old banker with nasal discharge, sneezing and a sensation of a blocked nose. His past medical history include asthma and eczema. He is otherwise fit and well and is on no regular medications.

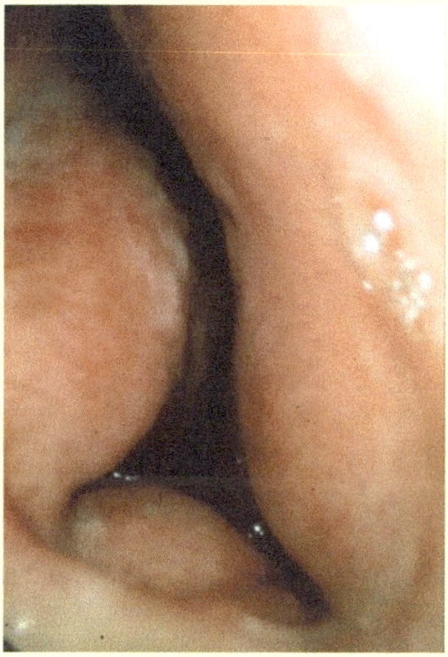

Figure 3.1.6 Rhinitis

Focusing question	Answer
What is the most likely diagnosis and what is the different aetiology?	• Rhinitis ○ Allergic ○ Non-allergic: e.g. infective, vasomotor/intrinsic (due to autonomic imbalance).
Management	**Answer**
What questions would you ask in the history?	• Symptoms: ○ Nasal discharge (rhinorrhoea). Characterise this discharge. ○ Nasal congestion ○ Sneezing • Ask about **R**hinorrhoea (and colour of discharge), **O**bstruction, **P**ain/pressure, **E**pistaxis, **S**mell, **I**tching, **S**neezing (ROPES IS) • History of atopy (asthma, eczema, hay fever) suggests allergic rhinitis. • Triggers: changes in temperature (vasomotor), allergens, chemicals. • Recent or recurrent URTIs can suggest infective causes. • Family History: Hereditary systemic causes.
How would you examine this patient?	• Anterior rhinoscopy/FNE: inflammation of mucosa, turbinate hypertrophy, nasal discharge (clear or mucopus).

What investigations could you order?	• Skin-prick tests or RAST if allergy is suspected • Blood tests to detect systemic or hereditary diseases. • Consider CT scan of nose and paranasal sinus if condition is not responding to treatment.

What would be the treatment plan?	• Conservative:
	    o Allergen avoidance in the case of allergic rhinosinusitis
	• Medical:
	    o Nasal decongestants such as Otrivine for the acute phase but avoid usage for more than 1 week as this can lead to rhinitis medicamentosa with long term use.
	    o Steroids: sprays, drops or oral steroids (eg mometasone).
	    o Antihistamines if allergic symptoms are present (sneezing and itching)
	    o Others: Montelukast (anti-leucotrienes) , sodium cromoglycate (mast cell stabiliser)
	• Consider antibiotic therapy (preferably macrolides) if primary or secondary bacterial infection is suspected
	• Consider reduction of turbinates (only considered if medical therapy is not controlling symtoms of allergic

	rhinosinusitis).

3.1.7 NASOPHARYNGEAL CARCINOMA

Clinical scenario
A 70-year old oriental gentleman presented with a 2month history of unilateral nasal obstruction and recurrent epistaxis, and facial pain with otalgia. Of note he also reports some recent weight loss. Examination of his nose reveal a unilateral nasal lesion.

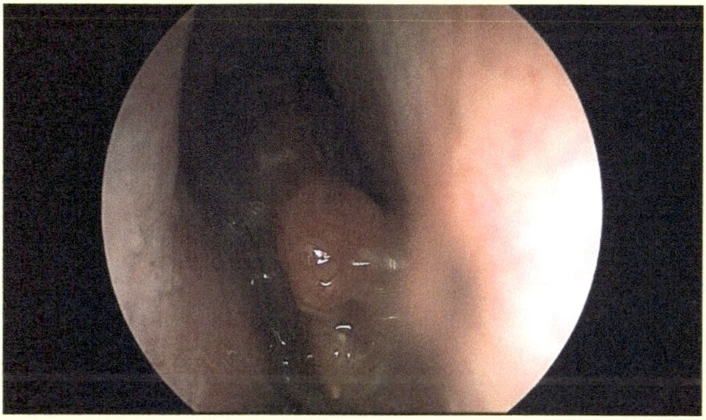

Figure 3.1.7. endoscopic examination of the nose showing the nasal lesion

Focusing question	Answer
What is the most likely diagnosis?	• Nasopharyngeal carcinoma (NPC)

Management	Answer
What are the most common symptoms?	• Nasal obstruction • Recurrent epistaxis • Reduced hearing. (Secondary to obstruction of Eustachian tube opening, causing ipsilateral middle ear effusion.) • Facial pain/referred otalgia • Note: Unilateral symptoms should always be treated with a high index of suspicion of a sinister pathology
How would you examine this patient?	• Full ENT and Head & Neck Examination o Include otoscopy • Flexible nasoendoscopy (visualise Fossa of Rosenmuller in particular)

What further investigations would you request?	• Audiometry & tympanometry
	• Imaging: CT/MRI
	• Tissue biopsy:
	  o Nasopharyngeal mass
	  o Fine needle aspiration/core or excision biopsy of lymph node if metastasis suspected.

Additional Question (s)	**Answer**
Name a risk factor for NPC	• Nitrosamines – found in salted fish, often consumed by oriental communities. • Associated with latent EBV – found in patients who develop NPC.

3.2 SINUSES

3.2.1 RHINOSINUSITIS

Clinical scenario

A 35-year-old woman who is generally fit and well presents with a 3 day history facial pain and pressure, and blocked nose. She has never had this before. She has recently been suffering from a flu-like illness. She is on no regular medications and has no allergies.

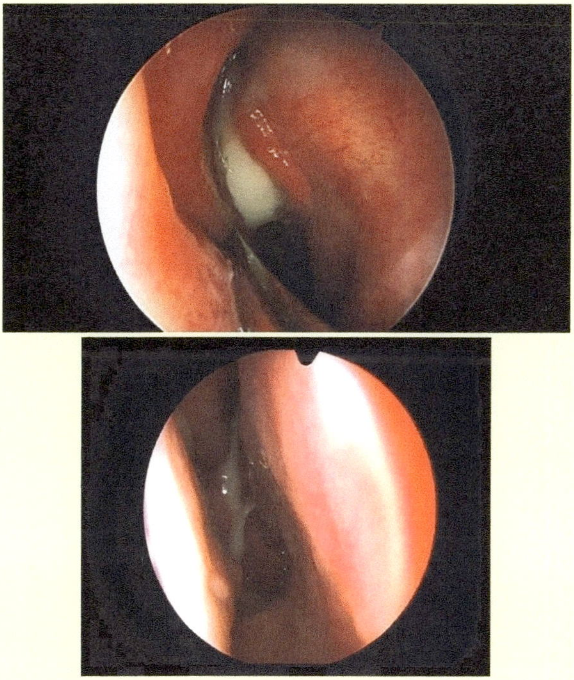

Figure 3.2.1a Acute rhinosinusitis (ARS) with pus arising from the left maxillary sinus.

Focusing question	Answer
What is the most likely diagnosis and the differential diagnoses?	• Acute rhinosinusitis (ARS) is the most likely diagnosis (NOTE that rhinosinusitis is the commonest condition in the world). • Chronic rhinosinusitis (CRS) • Nasal polyp • Sinonasal tumour • Neurological: Trigeminal neuralgia, migraine
Management	**Answer**
What questions would you ask in the history?	• Nasal discharge or blockage are the most important symptoms • Where exactly is the facial pain/pressure. Bifrontal and bimalar pressure is typical. Pain is uncommon in chronic rhinosinusitis (more common in acute sinusitis) • Anosmia. • Post-nasal drip • Duration of symptoms. If Sx <12 weeks, this is ARS. If Sx >12 weeks, this is CRS. • Recent upper respiratory tract infection • Ask about the symptoms of complications of rhinosinusitis (see below) • High temperature
How would you examine this patient?	• Inspection o Anterior rhinoscopy/flexible or rigid nasendoscopy. o Look specifically for pus, polyps, oedema, congestion of inferior turbinates.

How is rhinosinusitis diagnosed?	• The following answers are according to the EPOS (European Position Paper on Rhinosinusitis and Nasal Polyps) guidelines:
	• According to the EPOS (European position paper) guidelines:
	• ≥2 of the following symptoms:
	  o Must include one of: nasal obstruction, or nasal discharge
	  o +/- facial pain/pressure
	  o +/- reduction of loss smell
	• ARS = symptoms completely resolve within 12 weeks.
	• CRS = symptoms do not completely resolve within 12 weeks

How is its' severity graded?	• Through a Visual Analogue Scale (VAS) of Symptoms:
	  o Mild: VAS 0-3
	  o Moderate: VAS >3-7
	  o Severe: VAS >7-10

How is ARS managed?	• Symptoms <5 days: symptomatic relief only.
	• Symptoms persisting or increasing after 5 days:
	  o Moderate: intranasal steroids: If symptom improvement in 48 hours, continue for 7-14 days. If no improvement after 14 days, refer to ENT.
	  o Severe (severe facial pain or temp

	> 38^{0}C): intranasal steroids + oral antibiotics: - If symptom improvement in 48 hours, continue for 7-14 days. - If no improvement in 48 hours, refer to ENT.
How is CRS managed?	• No nasal polyps on examination o Mild: Topical steroids, nasal douche o No improvement after three months or moderate/severe: Topical steroids, nasal douche, culture, long-term antibiotics o No improvement: consider FESS • Nasal polyps present on examination o Mild: Topical steroid spray, nasal douche - Review after 3 months: - Improvement: Continue medications, review 6 monthly. - No improvement: Follow moderate pathway. o Moderate: Topical steroid spray (can increase dose or consider steroid drops), nasal douche, consider doxycycline - Review after 3 months: - Improvement: Continue topical steroid spray, nasal douche. Follow-up 6 monthly.. - No improvement: Consider CT

	scan +/- surgery (FESS) o Severe: Topical steroids, nasal douche, oral steroids (short course). - Improvement: Follow "Moderate" treatment pathway. - No improvement: Consider CT scan +/- surgery (FESS)
Additional Question (s)	**Answer**
What factors predispose to sinusitis?	• Local: upper respiratory tract infection, rhinitis, nasal polyps or tumours. • General: Immunosuppression, hereditary mucociliary disorders.
What are the complications of sinusitis?	• Orbital: periorbital cellulitis, orbital abscess • Intracranial: meningitis, encephalitis, intracranial abscess, cavernous sinus thrombosis • Local spread into bone - Osteomyelitis, e.g. Pott's Puffy Tumour
Describe the anatomy of the paranasal sinuses and the drainage system.	• 4 paired air-filled cavities: frontal, ethmoidal, maxillary, sphenoidal • Drainage system: o Maxillary sinus –middle meatus o Ethmoidal sinus –middle and superior meati o Sphenoidal sinus – sphenoethmoidal recess in the middle meatus

	○ Frontal sinus – infundibulum in the middle meatus

Other Relevant Clinical Photographs
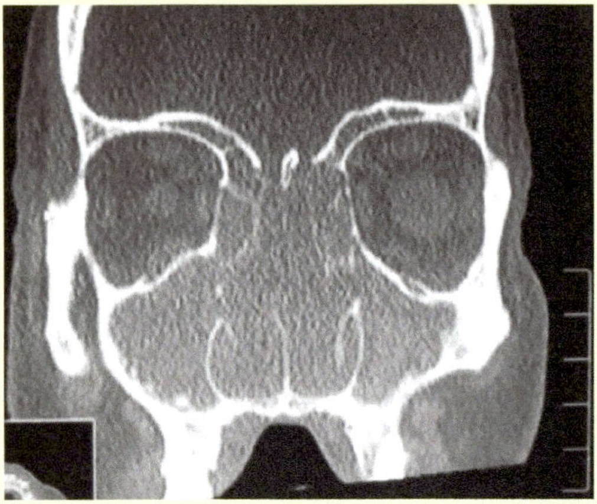 **Figure 3.2.1b.** CT coronal image showing pan-sinusitis secondary to nasal polyps.

3.2.2 PERIORBITAL CELLULITIS

Clinical scenario
A 20-year-old man presents with a unilateral oedematous and erythematous swelling around the left eye. He reports a recent stuffy nose and nasal blockage. He is currently on no medication, and is otherwise fit and well with no other concerns.

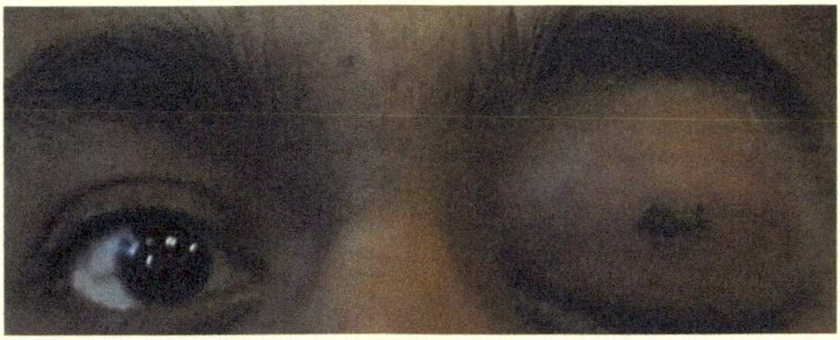

Figure 3.2.2. Periorbital cellulitis

Focusing question	Answer
What common condition often precedes orbital cellulitis?	• Rhinosinusitis • Other upper respiratory tract infections often precede the cellulitis.
Management	**Answer**
What questions would you ask in this patient?	• Swelling/redness of eyelid • Inability to open the eye • Changes in vision • Symptoms of upper respiratory tract infection and rhinosinusitis. • High temperature • Changes in colour vision • Swelling of eye **Note. Orbital abscess is an emergency as it can lead to blindness.**

On examination, what specific signs would you look for?	• Proptosis and chemosis • Conjunctival redness • Loss of colour vision • Opthalmoplegia
How would you investigate this patient?	• Flexible nasendoscopy for evidence of sinusitis • Bloods: markers of inflammation (WCC, CRP) blood cultures • Pus cultures • Imaging via CT head, paranasal sinus and orbit with contrast. (Consider imaging early if patients cannot be assessed appropriately, especially in children, to rule out orbital abscess).
How would you manage this patient?	• Joint admission between paediatrics, ENT and ophthalmology • Broad spectrum antibiotics • Nasal decongestant • Referral for urgent surgery (drainage of abscess) may be required. This can be done through an external approach and/or endoscopically.

Additional Question (s)	Answer
What is the difference between pre-septal and post-septal orbital cellulitis?	• Infection may be anterior or posterior to the orbital septum (this is different to the nasal septum). o Pre-septal = anterior to septum o Post-septal = posterior to septum (this is more commonly associated with sinusitis and poses a higher risk to vision)
What is the classification system used for orbital/periorbital cellulitis?	• Chandler's classification system

3.2.3 SINONASAL MALIGNANCY

Clinical scenario
A 70-year-old carpenter has presented to your ENT clinic. He complains of left side of the nose being blocked, and an increasing frequency of nose bleeds over the last month. He has never suffered from nosebleeds in the past. He has also noticed some weight loss in this period. He has a significant smoking history. Otherwise he is fit and well and is on no regular medications.

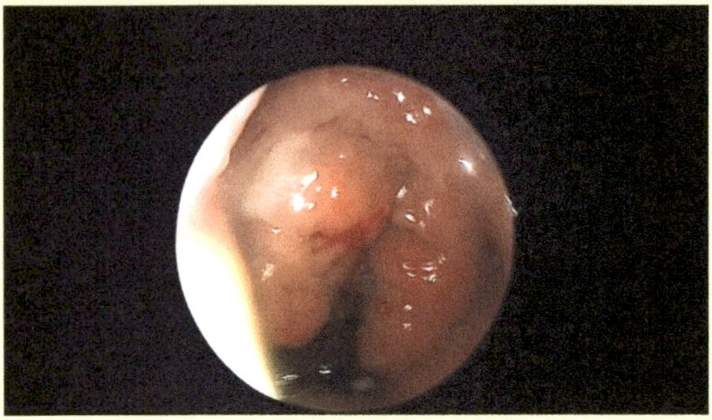

Figure 3.2.3. Endoscopic view of the nasal cavity showing a lesion in the post nasal space.

Focusing question	Answer
How would you classify the types of sinonasal tumour?	• Malignant o Squamous cell carcinoma o Adenocarcinoma • Benign: o Basal cell tumour o Papilloma o Osteoma

Management	Answer

What questions would you ask in this patient?	• Key nasal symptoms:
	  o Nasal obstruction/discharge, often unilateral.
	  o Epistaxis (often recurrent), often unilateral.
	  o Signs of local compression: Facial pain/swelling, visual disturbance, headaches.
	• Systemic symptoms:
	  o Weight loss
	  o Loss of appetite
	  o Night sweats
	• Social history- consider the risk factors.
	  o Occupation: exposure to wood dust (carpentry), nickel, textiles
	  o Smoking and alcohol intake
	Note: unilateral symptoms should always raise alarm bells for malignancy

How would you examine this patient?	• Perform full ENT, head and neck examination
	  o Otoscopy: look for unilateral middle ear effusion
	  o Neck: lymphadenopathy

What investigations should be carried out to help with staging and	• Flexible/rigid nasendoscopy
	• Radiological:
	  o CT sinuses, head, neck and chest
	  o MRI scan (better for soft tissue lesions)

grading of the tumour?	• Biopsy for histology • Staging = TNM

How would you manage this patient following staging?	• Multidisciplinary team approach
	  ○ Surgery
	  ○ Radiotherapy
	  ○ Chemotherapy
	  ○ Palliative

Chapter 4

Head, Neck and Throat

4.1 INFECTIVE

4.1.1 TONSILLITIS

Clinical scenario

A mother brings her 12-year-old child to see you. She states the child is refusing to eat due to a sore throat and is complaining of ear pain and fever over the last 3 days. The child has no other medical or surgical problems. You suspect acute tonsillitis.

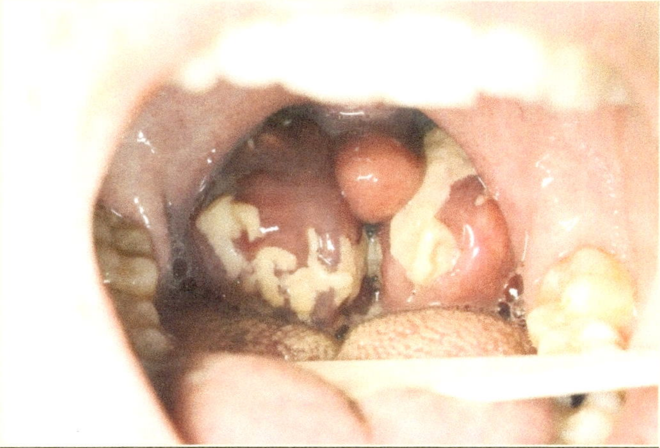

Fig 4.1.1. Bilateral tonsillitis

Focusing question	Answer
What are the possible aetiological agents of acute tonsillitis?	• Bacterial: *Streptococcus pyogenes, Streptococcus pneumonia, Haemophilus influenzae, Corynebacterium diphtheria* • Viral: Rhinovirus, adenovirus, Epstein-Barr virus
Management	**Answer**
What questions would you ask in this patient?	• Sore throat • Dysphagia ± odynophagia • Fever, malaise- a part of the "CENTOR score". The higher this score, the more likely the patient is to have bacterial tonsillitis. • Absence of cough- also a part of the "CENTOR score" • Ask about preceding upper or lower respiratory tract infections • Number of episodes of acute tonsillitis or quinsies (peritonsillar abscess) in the past. This is important for assessing their eligibility for surgery. • Any problems with breathing (airway obstruction or obstructive sleep apnoea) • Ask about whether the patient is able to drink. If not, they will require admission for intravenous fluids. • Psychosocial: impact of tonsillitis on daily life e.g. missing school, exams.

What signs would you look for on examination?	• Bilateral tonsil swelling. Asymmetrical tonsil swelling is worrying. This may suggest a peri-tonsillar abcess on one side, or an underlying malignancy. • Exudate/pus on tonsils may be present • Enlarged lymph nodes e.g. jugulodigastric node- Part of the "CENTOR score" • Pyrexia • Trismus • Noisy breathing
How would you investigate this patient?	• Microbiology: Throat swabs • Bloods e.g. FBC, Infectious Mononucleosis screen for Epstein-Barr virus. PCR is preferable to the monospot test.
How would you treat this patient?	• Supportive Measures e.g. encourage oral intake of fluids. Admit for intravenous fluids if cannot tolerate oral fluids. • Medical: analgesia, antipyrexials, IV steroids and antibiotics may be required as per hospital guidelines. Avoid amoxicillin or ampicillin as these can cause a rash in glandular fever (Epstein-Barr virus infection). • Surgical: referral to ENT specialists for tonsillectomy at a later date if they fit the criteria for tonsillectomy

	(tonsillectomy is not done when the tonsil is inflamed due to the increased risk of bleeding).
Additional Question (s)	**Answer**
Name 3 types of 'tonsils' found in the pharynx: What abscesses can occur following tonsillitis?	• Palatine tonsils - in the oropharynx • Pharyngeal/adenoids - in nasopharynx • Lingual tonsils - on posterior tongue • Peritonsillar abscess • Retropharyngeal abscess • Parapharyngeal abscess
What advice would you give specifically to patients who test positive for glandular fever	• Longer course of infection • Require initial liver function tests and repeated few weeks following discharge in community to ensure improvement. • Risk of splenic rupture - avoid significant physical activity or contact sports for at least 6 weeks. May require USS to confirm splenic size.

4.1.2 SUPERFICIAL NECK ABSCESS

Clinical scenario
A 3-year-old girl presents with a large tender swelling on the left side of her neck. The mother claims that the lump is red and warm, and that her daughter has recently spiked a fever.

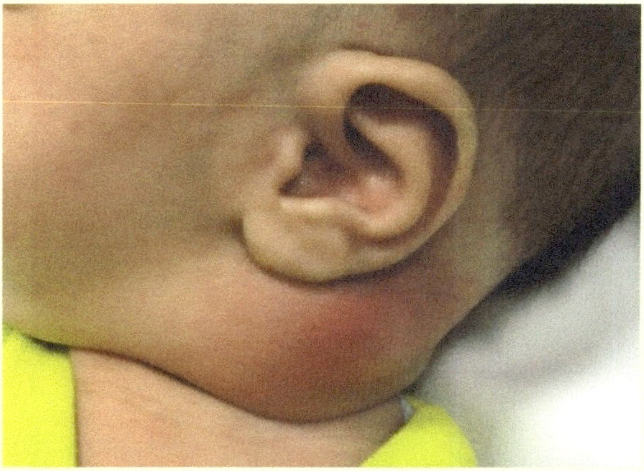

Figure 4.1.2 Intact superficial neck abscess in a baby.
(Image from ENT Tzar Urgent Care in Otolaryngology)

Focusing question	Answer
What is the likely diagnosis?	Intact superficial neck abscess
Management	**Answer**
What questions would you ask in this patient?	• Duration of the neck swelling? Has it changed in size or shape? • Was there any previous lump present? • Is there discharge from the lump? If so, what colour?

	• Systemic symptoms e.g. fever, malaise • Any recent history of illness or infections • History of: immunosuppression, TB
What features would you be looking for on examination?	• Site, size, shape, fluctuation, overlying skin colour • Temperature • Tenderness on palpation? • Visible discharge? • Lymphadenopathy • Systemic features e.g. pyrexia, tachycardia, hypotension
How would you investigate this patient?	• Ultrasound scan, to determine any suppuration and to guide possible incision and drainage. Also used as baseline (repeated if worsens) • Bloods e.g. FBC, inflammatory markers, blood culture • Swabs of discharge for culture and staining
How would you treat this patient?	• Admit patient • Provide analgesia and antibiotic as per hospital guidelines • Incision and drainage may be required

4.1.3 DEEP NECK SPACE INFECTIONS

Clinical scenario
A 4-year-old boy presents to you with high fevers, neck swelling and a reduced range of neck movement. The father informs you that his son has recently had an infection. There is no signs of meningitis, and the child is otherwise fit and well, and not on any medications at present.

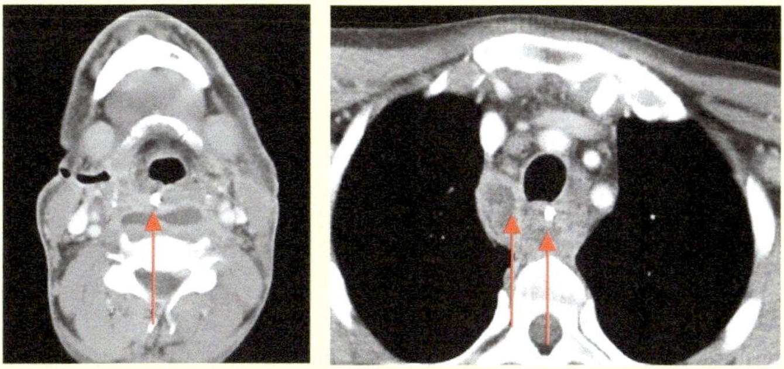

Figure 4.1.3 CT showing a deep neck space abscess with extension into the upper mediastinum.

(Image from ENT Tzar Urgent Care in Otolaryngology)

Focusing question	Answer
What common infections or factors precede deep neck space infections?	• Tonsillitis • Dental infection • Mastoiditis • Pharyngeal foreign body • Being immunocompromised

Management	Answer
What symptoms and features could you ask about in this patient?	• Painful neck and throat • Neck swelling or reduced neck movement • Dysphagia/Odynophagia • Change in voice • Stridor, noisy breathing and drooling • Fever • Recent infections, or past drug history • Ask about the preceding, predisposing infections (see above)

How would you examine this patient?	• Initial assessment of patient should be focussed on the airway, breathing and circulation status.
	    o The airway may be compromised from the mass effect of any swelling or abscess
	    o Circulation may be affected due to sepsis
	    o Hence senior help and anaesthetic assessment is often urgently required
	• Examine neck for swelling or masses
	• Trismus
	• Marked tenderness on cervical rotation
	• Flexible nasendoscopy can visualise extent of airway compromise and to identify bulging of pharyngeal wall

How would you investigate this patient?	• Bloods e.g. FBC, inflammatory markers, blood cultures • Lateral soft tissue neck x-ray ± orthopantomogram (OPG) if dental cause suspected • CT neck/thorax with contrast to determine the nature of the infection/abscess, as well as site and causes.
How would you treat this patient?	• Make sure the airway is secured early (this may require intubation, or tracheostomy) • IV broad spectrum antibiotics as per hospital protocol and discussion with microbiologist • Surgical incision and drainage may be required if no response to antibiotics or if significant abscess.
Additional Question (s)	**Answer**
What types of neck space infections do you know of?	• Retropharyngeal abscess • Parapharyngeal abscess
What are possible complications of deep neck space infections?	• Mediastinitis • Vascular: Mycotic carotid aneurysm, internal jugular vein thrombosis

4.1.4 HEAD AND NECK TUBERCULOSIS

Clinical scenario

35-year-old male presents to you with a non-tender mass of the neck, which you suspect to be a lymph node. The mass has been enlarging over the period of 4-6 months, and the patient has complained of general malaise and fever. On further exploration, you note a positive HIV status. He is a non-smoker.

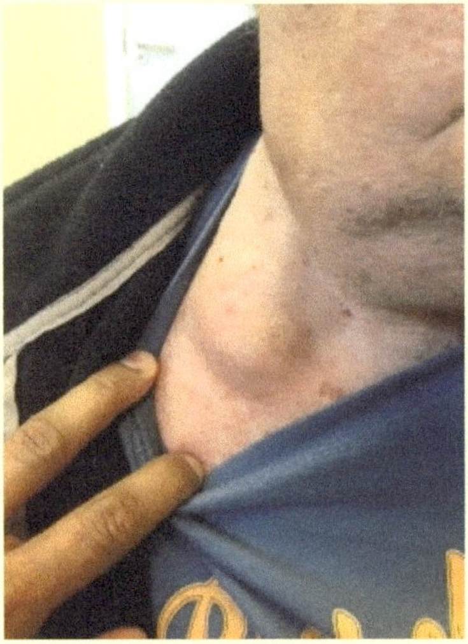

Figure 4.1.4 Cervical lymphadenopathy associated with TB

Focusing question	Answer
What is the likely diagnosis? Why is this patient more prone to this disease?	• Cervical lymphadenitis due to TB ('scrofula') • More prone in immunocompromised status, e.g. secondary to HIV
What are other possible differentials for this presentation?	• Acute reactive lymph nodes/ abscesses • Lymphoma • Malignancy and metastasis from head and neck squamous cell carcinoma

Management	Answer
What questions would you ask in this patient?	• Duration, onset • Progression: changes in the lump • Recent infections e.g. tonsillitis • Systemic features: fever, weight loss, night sweats, malaise, pruritus • Past Medical history of being immunocompromised or having opportunistic infections
How would you examine this patient?	• Focussed neck lump examination • General examination: weight loss, pyrexia

What possible diagnostic investigations could you request for this patient?	• Ultrasound scan with fine needle aspiration and cytology (FNAC) • Excision biopsy for pathology if FNAC results are not conclusive • Culture and Ziehl-Neelsen stain for acid fast bacteria
How would you treat this patient?	• Multidrug therapy is e.g. rifampicin, isoniazid, pyrazinamide, ethambutol • It is also important to note that TB is a notifiable disease and that contact tracing is often required.
Additional Question (s)	**Answer**
What is the aetiological agent responsible for TB?	• Mycobacterium Tuberculosis
What other systems does TB affect?	• TB can affect any organ system, in particular: o Pulmonary o Central nervous system o Renal and adrenal glands o Musculoskeletal system

What characteristic pathological finding under the microscope is associated with TB?	• Caseating granuloma (type iv hypersensivity reaction)

4.2 NON-INFECTIVE

4.2.1 AIRWAY OBSTRUCTION

Clinical scenario
An 80-year-old lady presented with noisy breathing. She had no other significant past medical history and was on no regular medications. On examination stridor was evident and she was in obvious distress.

Focusing question	Answer

How can airway obstruction be classified?	• **Airway Obstruction:**
	  o **Upper** airway obstruction = above larynx
	  o **Lower** airway obstruction = below larynx

Management	**Answer**

How would you examine this patient and what specific signs would you look for?	• LOOK for signs of respiratory distress:
	  o Central cyanosis
	  o Difficulty in speaking sentences
	  o Use of accessory muscles of respiration
	  o Observations: High respiratory rate, low oxygen saturations
	• LISTEN for noises of airway obstruction:
	  o **Stridor**: high-pitched, inspiratory (can be biphasic)
	    ▪ Indicates obstruction at or below larynx
	  o **Stertor:** low-pitched, inspiratory. Sounds like snoring.

	▪ Indicates obstruction *above* larynx. Usually soft palate/pharynx. • Full ENT examination including FNE to identify area of obstruction
How would you manage this patient?	**This is an emergency. Call for help (Anaesthetics and ENT are essential)** **1. Initial Resuscitation – airway management:** • High flow oxygen or Heliox (mixture of helium + adrenaline) • Basic airway manoeuvres (head tilt, chin lift, jaw thrust). • Suction any fluids- secretions, etc. if appropriate. • Airway adjuncts: o Oropharyngeal o Nasopharyngeal (avoid if basal skull fracture suspected) • Nebulized adrenaline • Endotracheal intubation to secure the airway. • Surgical airway (a last resort): - Cricothyroidotomy - Emergency tracheostomy **2. Treatment of specific cause if identified early:** • Depends on aetiology: refer to table below **3. Further investigations:** • Imaging:

	<ul><li><ul><li>Lateral soft tissue neck X-Ray (e.g. significant soft tissue swelling, foreign body)</li><li>Chest X-Ray. May show radio-opaque foreign bodies or signs of aspiration pneumonia.</li><li>CT/MRI of neck</li></ul></li><li>Direct visualisation, especially if foreign body is suspected in theatre (laryngoscopy, pharyngoscopy, bronchoscopy)</li></ul>

Additional Question (s)	Answer

Name some causes of airway obstruction.	Always **classify** when answering these questions. (Note: these are not all the causes – the list would be too long)
	Upper airway:
	• Congenital:
	  o Choanal atresia
	  o Craniofacial malformations (e.g. microagnathisma, macroglossia.)
	• Acquired:
	  o Anaphylaxis (usually treated medically and no ENT input is required unless airway becomes compromised)
	  o Foreign Body
	  o Trauma
	  o Epiglottitis
	  o Deep neck abscess
	  o Neoplasia
	
	Lower airway:
	• Congenital:
	  o Laryngomalacia
	  o Tracheomalacia
	
	• Acquired:
	  o Foreign body
	  o Trauma
	  o Infection: Croup (Laryngotracheobronchitis)

Diagnosis and Management of Specific Causes of Airway Obstruction	
Peritonsillar Abscess (Quinsy)	• Clinical signs: Trismus, muffled ("hot potato") speech, pyrexia • Management: Aspiration/Incision, IV Antibiotics and Steroids.
Epiglottitis	• Clinical signs: Recent URTI, Pyrexia, drooling. "Tripod" posture. • Management: Do not attempt examination or any invasive tests– this may compromise the airway as the child is likely to be distressed. o Call for help: anaesthetist and ENT o Protect airway – maintain upright posture. o Transfer to safe area (operating theatre) o Direct laryngoscopy +/- intubation o IV antibiotics, fluids **once airway secure**
Croup	• Clinical signs: Stridor, barking cough • Management: Maintain airway, dexamethasone, antibiotics
Ludwig's Angina (Submandibular space infection)	• Often follows dental infection or tonsillitis • Clinical signs: Trismus, swelling in floor of mouth • Imaging (ultrasound/CT) is often required to identify extent of disease

	• Management: IV antibiotics, Aspiration or I&D under GA.
Anaphylaxis	• Clinical signs: Urticaria, Respiratory distress. • Adult Mx: Adrenaline 0.5ml of 1:1000 IM, Hydrocortisone 200mg IV), chlorphenamine 10mg IV. Management and doses may vary for different hospitals and for children.

4.2.2 GASTRO-OESOPHAGEAL REFLUX DISEASE (GORD) and LARYNGOPHARYNGEAL REFLUX (LPR)

Clinical scenario

A 45-year-old overweight gentleman presents worsening pain after eating. He complains of a dry cough particularly at night for over 6 months. Sometimes his voice feels sore and hoarse for no apparent reason. It is particularly worse after spicy foods, drinking alcohol and coffee. He has suffered no weight loss or night sweats. He has no other past medical history but has a 20-pack year history of smoking.

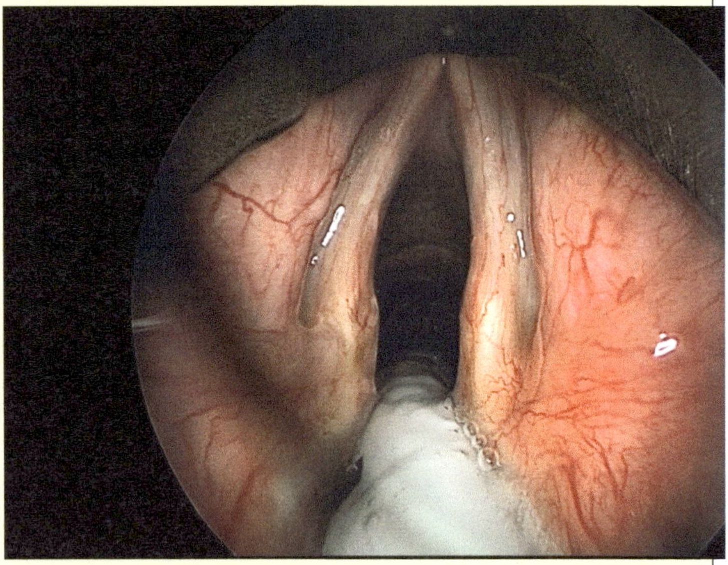

Figure 4.2.2 Endoscopic view of a larynx showing increased vascularity secondary to chronic cough associated with GORD

Focusing question	Answer
What is the most likely diagnosis and what are the differential diagnoses?	• Most likely: Gastro-oesophageal reflux disease (GORD) • Peptic ulcer disease • Oesophageal/gastric carcinoma
Management	**Answer**
What symptoms would you ask the patient?	• Heartburn • Water brash • Dysphagia/odynophagia • Hoarse voice • Onset of symptoms: after spicy foods, worse at night (due to position) • Red flags: weight loss, iron deficiency anaemia/GI bleeding, mass • Family History
How would you examine this patient?	• Full ENT and Head & Neck examination • Flexible nasendoscopy: looking for inflammation around the vocal cords and larynx, consistent with laryngopharyngeal reflux.
What possible investigations would you consider this patient?	• Blood tests: Iron deficiency anaemia • Radiology: Barium swallow if suspicion of a sliding hiatus hernia is high. • Direct visualisation: OGD (endoscopy) may show evidence of oesophagitis, Barrett's oesophagus, gastritis, ulcers, cancer.

	• Specialist tests:
	  o 24 hour pH monitoring is the gold standard for diagnosis of GORD.
	  o H.pylori testing. E.g. urease breath test.

How would you treat this patient?	• Conservative: Often effective in itself.
	  o Stop smoking, alcohol
	  o Avoid spicy, fatty foods, caffeine
	• Medical
	  o Antacid medication
	  o Proton pump inhibitor, e.g. omeprazole
	  o H2 receptor antagonists such as ranitidine.
	  o H.pylori eradication therapy.
	• Surgery: Nissen's fundoplication- if patient has severe symptoms, confirmed GORD and is refractory to medical therapy.

4.2.3 PHARYNGEAL POUCH

Clinical scenario

A 75-year-old man presents with a 3-month history of regurgitation and halitosis. He also mentions progressive dysphagia. He is otherwise fit and well, and reports no weight loss.

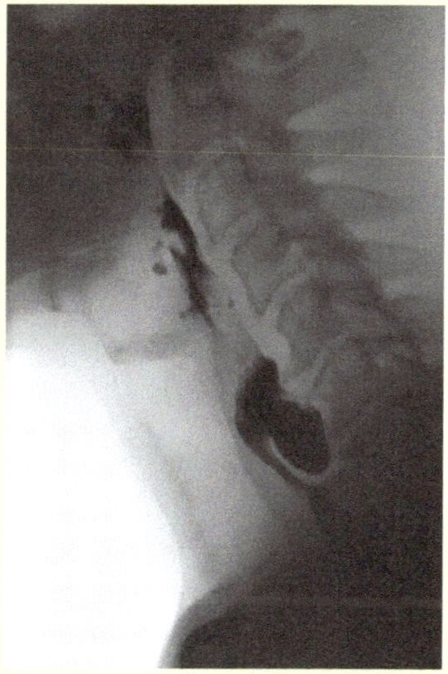

Fig 4.2.3. Barium swallow demonstrating a pharyngeal pouch.

Focusing question	Answer
What is the most likely diagnosis?	• Pharyngeal Pouch
Can you name some other causes of dysphagia?	• Gastrointestinal: Benign oesophageal strictures, achalasia, Pharyngeal/oesophageal/gastric cancer.

	• Neurological: Myasthenia gravis, multiple sclerosis • Others: Systemic sclerosis, Plummer-Vinson syndrome
Management	**Answer**
What symptoms would you ask in this patient?	• Progressively worsening dysphagia • Halitosis • Regurgitation • Neck lumps • Cough (aspiration) • Red Flags and systemic features e.g. weight loss, night sweats to rule out malignancy
How would you examine this patient?	• Full Head and Neck examination including FNE. • Full cranial and peripheral nerve examination • Abdominal examination
What investigations may you consider ordering?	• Contrast swallow (e.g. barium swallow) • Chest X-Ray (patients are at an increased risk of aspiration pneumonia) • OGD (endoscopy) – to rule out other causes of symptoms (however, there is a risk of perforation)
How would you treat this patient?	• Conservative (usually if the pouch is small and asymptomatic, or patient

	has significant comorbidities) • Medical botulinum toxin injection into cricopharyngeus • Surgery: repair can be carried out as an endoscopic stapling or open procedure 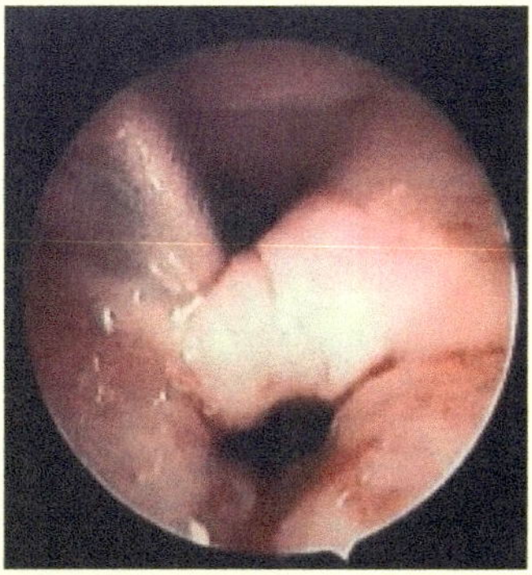 **Figure 4.2.3a** endoscopic view of the osesophagus (with the metal sucker inside), cricopharyngeus bar and the opening of the pouch. 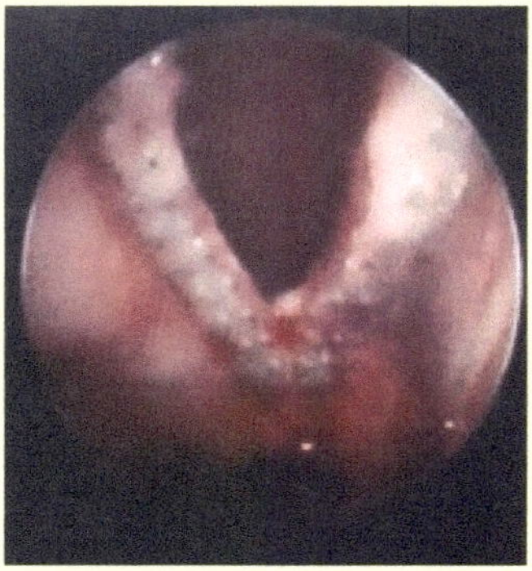 **Figure 4.2.3b** Cricopharyngeus muscle bar divided with a staple gun

Additional Question (s)	Answer
What muscles are responsible for constriction of the pharynx?	• The superior, middle and inferior constrictors. o Supplied by the pharyngeal plexus (CN IX, X) via the pharyngeal branch of CN X.
What is the pathophysiology of pharyngeal pouch?	• Increased pressure within the pharynx causes its mucosa to herniate through an area of weakness between the fibres of the inferior constrictor (between cricopharyngeus and thyropharyngeus), known as Killian's dehiscence.

4.2.4 VOICE DISORDERS

Clinical scenario
A 24-year-old opera singer presents with a 4-week history of a hoarse voice. She is particularly concerned as she is unable to work with the change in her voice. She is a smoker of 5 pack years, drinks very little alcohol. She has asthma and uses inhailers. Endoscopic view of her larynx reveal whitish patches.

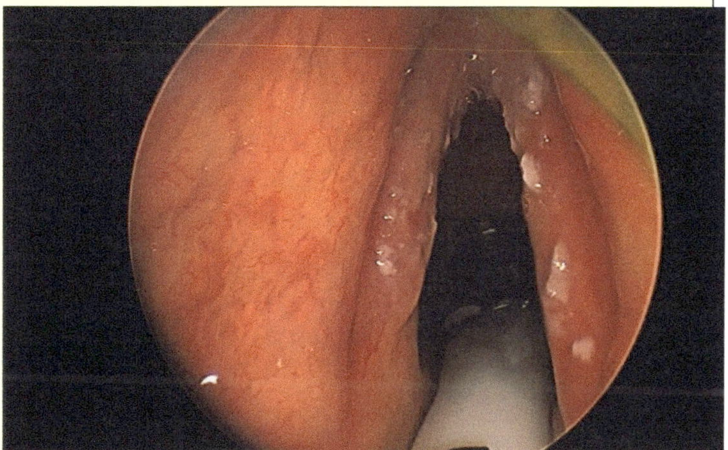

Figure 4.2.4a Endoscopic view of the fungus on larynx

Focusing question	Answer
What are the differential diagnoses?	Benign • Vocal cord nodules • Reinke's oedema • Vocal cord granulomas • Vocal cord polyps • Laryngeal papillomatosis

	• Infection such as fungus, especially if steroid inhalers are used Malignant • Laryngeal carcinoma
Management	**Answer**
What salient points would you address in the history?	• Hoarse voice o Duration o Progress: Is it improving or worsening o Any obvious causative factors? ▪ Previous surgery, including intubation ▪ Trauma • Difficulty breathing or swallowing • Symptoms of causative factors: GORD/LPR, rhinitis/sinusitis • Occupation: increased use of voice (singers) • Rule out red flags
How would you examine and investigate this patient?	• General ENT examination, including FNE. • Videostroboscopy - video designed to allow assessment of vocal cord movement on playback.
Common Voice Disorders and Clinical Details	
Vocal cord nodules	• History: Affects those who use their voice significantly, e.g. teachers, singers. • Examination: White lesions on vocal cords bilaterally, usually at the junction between the anterior 1/3 and middle 1/3. • Management: Speech rehabilitation

	(first-line), surgery
Vocal cord polyps	• History: Smokers, significant voice use • Examination: Unilateral lesions (vs. vocal cord nodules) • Management: Surgery
Reinke's oedema	• History: Smokers, more common in females, gastro-oesophageal reflux, affects those who use their voice significantly • O/E: Swelling of vocal cords (most commonly bilateral) • Management: Stop smoking, anti-reflux medication, speech rehabilitation, (surgery only considered if this is unhelpful)
Vocal process granulomas	• History: Gastro-oesophageal reflux, previous intubation, more common in males. • Examination: Lesions posteriorly (unilateral or bilateral) • Management: Speech rehabilitation, anti-reflux medication, surgery

<table>
<tr>
<td>Laryngeal papillomatosis</td>
<td>
<ul>
<li>Aetiology: Human Papillomavirus (most commonly HPV 6, 11)</li>
<li>History: Dysphonia, airway obstruction</li>
<li>Mx: Surgery (often using laser)</li>
</ul>
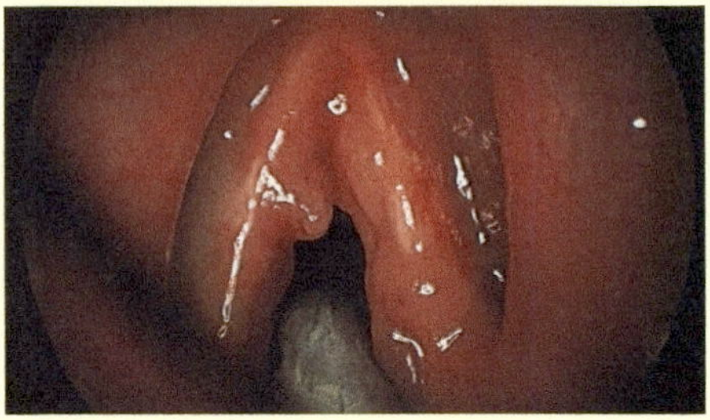

Figure 4.2.4. Endoscopic view of larynx showing laryngeal papillomatosis
</td>
</tr>
</table>

4.2.5 BENIGN SALIVARY GLAND DISEASE

Clinical scenario

A 60-year-old man presented with a painful swelling in the left side of her face that has increased in size over the last 2 months, and enlarges in size whilst she is eating. He is otherwise fit and well. He takes no regular medications. On examination you notice a unilateral swelling on his face.

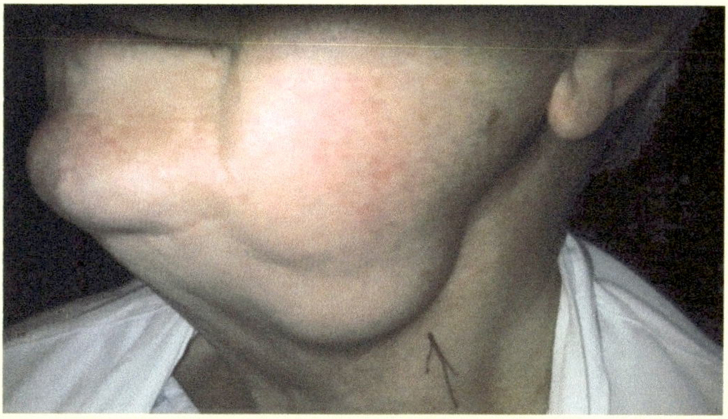

Figure 4.2.5 Clinical photograph of a left submandibular swelling

Focusing question	Answer
What are the main salivary glands?	• Parotid gland • Submandibular gland • Sublingual gland(s)

<table>
<tr><th>Management</th><th>Answer</th></tr>
<tr><td>What would you address in the history?</td><td><ul><li>Onset (sudden vs. gradual), duration</li><li>Progressive features</li><li>Unilateral (e.g. neoplasm) vs bilateral (e.g Mumps)</li><li>Swelling increases by eating (suggests parotitis or salivary stones)</li><li>Systemic symptoms – weight loss, night sweats (suggests malignancy)</li></ul></td></tr>
<tr><td>How would you examine this patient?</td><td><ul><li>Full ENT, Head & Neck Examination</li><li>Inspect: Unilateral, vs. bilateral, signs of infection/inflammation,<ul><li>Note: Test facial nerve for parotid swellings – weakness suggests infiltration by malignant cause.</li></ul></li><li>Palpate all salivary glands and neck lymph nodes<ul><li>Bimanual palpation – may detect calculi.</li><li>If parotitis, pus may be found and drained from parotid duct (opposite second upper molar).</li></ul></li></ul></td></tr>
<tr><td>What possible investigations could you request for this patient?</td><td><ul><li>Blood tests: WCC, CRP, autoimmune tests (Sjogren's syndrome)</li><li>Radiology:<ul><li>Ultrasound</li><li>Sialogram</li><li>MRI – if neoplastic cause suspected</li></ul></li><li>Biopsy (FNA or core) – if malignancy suspected. (Can be US-guided.)</li></ul></td></tr>
</table>

Additional Question (s)	Answer
Name some of the causes of salivary gland disease	Infective: • Mumps • Sialadenitis Inflammatory • Sjogren's syndrome Neoplastic: • Benign: Pleomorphic adenoma, Warthin's tumour • Malignant: these can be primary or secondary. Squamous cell carcinoma, adenocarcinoma, adenoid cystic carcinoma.

What are the most common benign salivary gland tumours?	**Pleomorphic adenoma**
	• Most common tumour of parotid.
	• Middle-aged population
	• History: Painless lump behind angle of jaw, progressively increases in size. Doesn't involve the facial nerve.
	• This is a benign growth but has a 10-15% chance of becoming malignant.
	• Key investigations:
	    o Radiology: US/MRI
	    o Tissue sample: FNA/Core biopsy
	• Management: Surgery: can recur if incomplete excision
	    o Risk of facial nerve damage

	Warthin's tumour/adenolymphoma
	• PC: Painless lump behind angle of jaw Bilateral in approximately 10-15% of cases
	• Key investigations:
	  ○ Radiology: US/MRI
	  ○ Tissue sample: FNA/Core biopsy
	• Management:
	  ○ Conservative: if patient elderly and non-symptomatic, and co-morbidity.
	  ○ Surgical: parotidectomy

4.2.6 THYROID DISEASE (BENIGN and MALIGNANT)

Clinical scenario
A 40-year-old lady presents with a neck swelling that has been increasing for over 2 years. He is concerned that it is slowly growing and that it is becoming more noticeable. On further questioning he reports diffculty swallowing and breathing. On examination he has a noticeable fullness in the front of her neck which moves up on swallowing. The CT scan of his neck is shown below

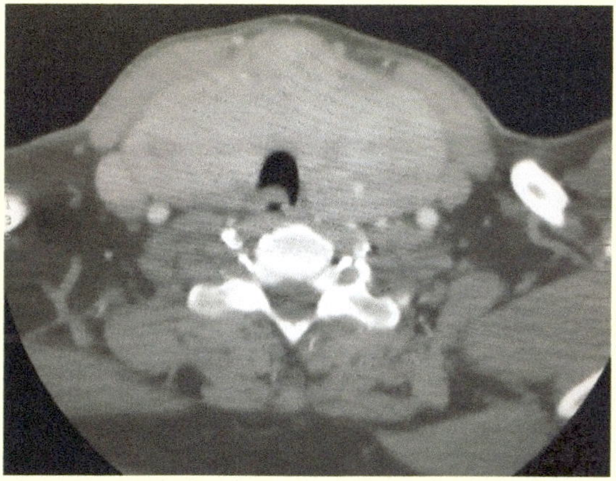

Figure 4.2.6a CT image of the neck through the thyroid gland

Focusing question	Answer

What do you think is the most likely diagnosis and what is in	• Most likely: Thyroid goitre with signs of thyrotoxicosis - Grave's disease
	• Differential diagnosis:
	  ○ Benign:
	    ▪ Thyroglossal cyst

your differential?	▪ Toxic goitre (associated with thyrotoxicosis) 1. Graves Disease 2. Toxic multinodular goitre 3. Toxic adenoma • Hashimoto's thyroiditis. In the early stage, this can present with thyrotoxicosis "Hashitoxicosis". o Malignant: 4 main types and lymphoma. ▪ Papillary. Is the most common thyroid cancer. ▪ Follicular ▪ Medullary ▪ Anaplastic ▪ Lymphoma
Management	**Answer**
What questions would you ask in the history?	• Duration, progressive symptoms • Systemically hypothyroid vs. hyperthyroid vs euthyroid. • Symptoms of external compression on surrounding structures: Dysphagia, difficulty breathing. • Systemic symptoms suggestive of malignancy: weight loss, night sweats. • Radiation exposure.

How would you examine this patient?	• Full general ENT, Head & Neck Examination including FNE. (Refer to Examinations chapter for comprehensive examination of neck lumps) • Systemic signs of hyper/hypothyroidism.

What investigations could you order?	• Blood tests:
	  ○ Thyroid function tests including thyroid auto-antibodies.
	• Radiology:
	  ○ Chest X-Ray: Tracheal deviation. Uncommonly done.
	  ○ Ultrasound
	  ○ CT/MRI – if neoplastic cause suspected
	  ○ Radio-iodine uptake test. Uncommonly performed these days. May be performed if trying to identify singular toxic nodule in a multinodular goitre.
	  ○ Radioisotope imaging, e.g. PET scan (usually once neoplasm confirmed)
	• Tissue sample for histology:
	  ○ FNA/Core Biopsy

Additional Question (s)	Answer	
What are the common benign thyroid lumps?	**Thyroglossal cyst**	• Persistent thyroglossal duct (embryologically this allows the descent of thyroid gland from the foramen caecum at the base of tongue). • Midline lump moves upwards on swallowing and tongue protrusion. Usually asymptomatic. • Investigations: Ultrasound, FNA. US is required to identify thyroid gland present. Occasionally the ectopic thyroid tissue in the thyroglossal cyst is the only thyroid tissue, and removal would cause hypothyroidism. • Management: Surgery - Sistrunk's procedure.

<table>
<tr>
<td></td>
<td></td>
<td>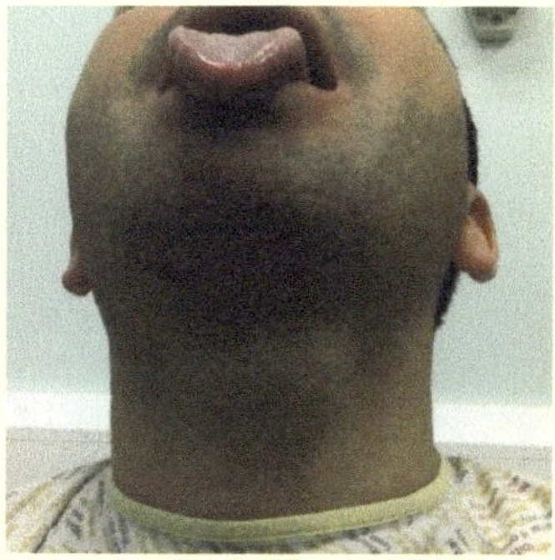
Figure 4.2.6b Large thyroglossal duct cyst (moves up on tongue protrusion)</td>
</tr>
<tr>
<td></td>
<td>Multinodular goitre</td>
<td>
<ul>
<li>Unknown aetiology. Areas of hyperplasia of thyroid gland, as well as atrophic areas.</li>
<li>Associated with iodine deficiency</li>
<li>Usually one lobe or nodule predominates. Can become large enough to cause compressive symptoms.</li>
<li>Investigations
<ul>
<li>Tissue sample: FNA/Core Biopsy</li>
<li>Imaging: US/CT (if features suggest external compression)</li>
</ul>
</li>
<li>Mx: Surgical excision</li>
</ul>
</td>
</tr>
</table>

		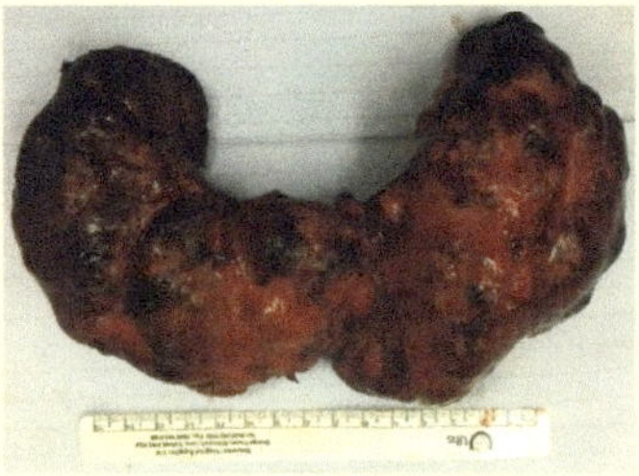 **Figure 4.2.6c** Large multinodular goitre

	Grave's disease	• Autoimmune cause – stimulatory anti-TSH antibodies.
		• Smooth neck lump (vs benign multinodular goitre)
		• Signs of hyperthyroidism:
		    o Note. Signs of thyroid eye disease: proptosis, exophthalmos, dry gritty eyes
		• Management:
		    o Medical: carbimazole, propylthiouracil, propranolol.
		    o Radioactive iodine (contraindicated in pregnancy)
		    o Rarely surgical excision if

		medically refractory, or compression symptoms. • Other thyroid lumps associated with thyrotoxicosis: o Toxic adenoma

	Hashimoto's Thyroiditis	• Autoimmune – anti-TPO (thyroid peroxidase) antibodies
		• Initially some patients present with hyperthyroidism (Hashitoxicosis), and later hypothyroidism.
		• Management:
		  o Conservative
		  o Medical: Thyroxine replacement
		  o Surgical excision (rarely required) – considered if medically refractory or compressive symptoms.
		• Note. Associated with thyroid lymphoma

<table>
<tr><td rowspan="2">What are the common malignant thyroid lumps?</td><td>Papillary Carcinoma</td><td><ul><li>Most common (approx. 60-80%)</li><li>Histology: “Orphan Annie nuclei”, “psammoma bodies”</li><li>Metastases via lymphatics.</li><li>Management:<ul><li>Surgical excision</li><li>Radioiodine</li><li>Long-term TSH suppression (with thyroxine)</li></ul></li></ul></td></tr>
<tr><td>Follicular Carcinoma</td><td><ul><li>2nd most common - approx. 15-20%</li><li>Associated with iodine deficiency</li><li>Haematogenous spread (cf papillary carcinoma)</li><li>Management:<ul><li>Surgical excision</li><li>Radioiodine</li><li>Monitor for recurrence with thyroglobulin.</li></ul></li><li>Note. Follicular carcinoma cannot be differentiated from follicular adenoma through FNA – thyroid lobectomy is required for diagnosis</li></ul></td></tr>
</table>

<table>
<tr><td></td><td>Medullary Carcinoma</td><td><ul><li>5-15%</li><li>Arises from the parafollicular cells.</li><li>Variety of paraneoplastic phenomena.</li><li>Associated with Multiple Endocrine Neoplasia Type II (MENII) Syndrome in small proportion.</li><li>Diagnosis:<ul><li>Tissue sample: FNA/Core biopsy</li><li>Imaging: US/CT</li><li>Elevated calcitonin is characteristic.</li></ul></li><li>Management:<ul><li>Surgical excision</li></ul></li></ul></td></tr>
<tr><td></td><td>Anaplastic Carcinoma</td><td><ul><li>Rare, primarily affects elderly</li><li>Increases in size quickly, and can cause signs of external compression</li><li>Diagnosis:<ul><li>Tissue sample: FNA/Core biopsy</li><li>Imaging: CT/MRI</li></ul></li><li>Management:<ul><li>Most palliative, which includes surgery.</li><li>Radiotherapy</li></ul></li></ul></td></tr>
</table>

		• Poor prognosis
	Lymphoma	• 5-10%. • Typically MALT lymphoma. • Associated with Hashimoto's thyroiditis and ionising radiation to the head and neck. • Management: Chemoradiotherapy

4.2.7 LARYNGEAL MALIGNANCY

Clinical scenario
A 60-year-old publican presents with a 12-week history of hoarseness in his voice. He also has dysphagia and has noticed some weight loss. Of note he has a 60-pack year history of smoking. An endoscopic view of his larynx is shown below.

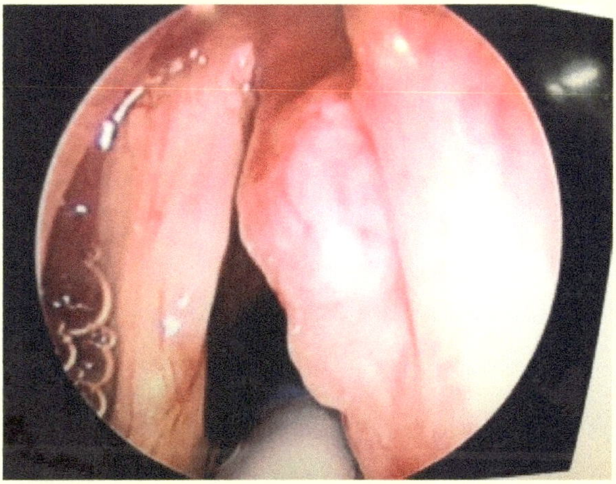

Figure 4.2.7 Laryngeal cancer of the left vocal cord

Focusing question	Answer
What is the suspected diagnosis?	• Laryngeal Cancer
Management	**Answer**
What questions would you ask in the history?	• Symptoms: o Persistent voice hoarseness o Dysphagia/odynophagia

	◦ Difficulty breathing ◦ Otalgia (referred pain) ◦ Systemic symptoms: weight loss, night sweats • Risk factors: ◦ Male ◦ Smoking, alcohol ◦ GORD/LPR
How would you examine this patient?	• Full ENT, Head & Neck Examination including FNE
How would you investigate this patient?	• Direct visualisation + take biopsies: Microlaryngoscopy, panendoscopy • Radiology: ◦ CT/MRI of neck ◦ Staging CT: Thorax, abdomen, pelvis
What modalities of treatment could be considered?	• Radiotherapy • Surgery: ◦ Laser surgery ◦ Laryngectomy +/- Neck dissection (for removal of nodes) • Chemotherapy
Additional Question (s)	**Answer**
How is this cancer staged?	**TNM:** • Tumour: Extent of local invasion • Node: Spread to lymph nodes • Metastasis: Extent of distant spread

What are the different sites of laryngeal cancer?	• Supraglottis (above level of larynx): 40-50% • Glottis: 50-60% • Subglottis: Approx 10%
What is the most common type of laryngeal cancer?	• Squamous cell carcinoma
What is the 5-year prognosis?	• Ranges from 50% (Stage 4) to approx. 90% (Stage 1). • Note. Functional outcomes (speech and swallow) are often poor

4.3 SURGICAL PROCEDURES

4.3.1 TRACHEOSTOMIES

Clinical Pictures

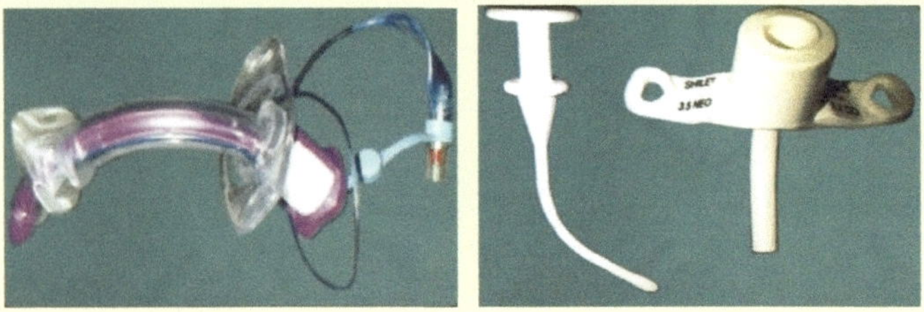

Fig 4.3.1: Cuffed adult tracheostomy and neonatal tracheostomy tubes.

Focusing question	Answer

What are indications for tracheostomy?	• Airway obstruction – as an emergency operation
	• Airway protection – often as an elective procedure
	  o Prior to major head & neck surgery
	  o Patients with neurological conditions
	• Ventilatory support – often electively for patients in in intensive care

Can you describe the operative procedure?	• Make incision through the following layers of the neck: skin, subcutaneous tissue, superficial cervical fascia (including platysma) and deep cervical fascia • Divide strap muscles and thyroid isthmus

	• Make vertical incision (or window) in trachea at approximately 2nd-4th tracheal ring • Tracheostomy tube inserted as endotracheal tube withdrawn by anaesthetist.

Can you name some complications?	• Immediate (≤24 hours post-op)
	    o Primary haemorrhage
	    o Damage to surrounding structures: recurrent laryngeal nerve palsy, oesophageal perforation
	• Early (1-14 days post-op)
	    o Secondary haemorrhage
	    o Tube dislodgement/obstruction
	• Late (> 14 days post-op)
	    o Tracheal stenosis
	    o Tracheocutaneous fistula

What the different types of tracheostomy tubes?	**Cuffed vs. non-cuffed tubes**
	• Advantages of cuff:
	    o Good for airway protection as it helps prevent aspiration/ respiratory secretions from leaking around tube.
	    o Useful for positive pressure ventilation.
	• Disadvantages of cuff:
	    o Reduced lumen diameter for airflow.

	Fenestrated tubes • Useful for speech • But not protective of lower respiratory tract from secretions **Tubes with inner tubes** • Useful for long-term tracheostomies as inner tubes can be removed regularly for cleaning.

4.3.2 LARYNGECTOMY

Clinical Pictures

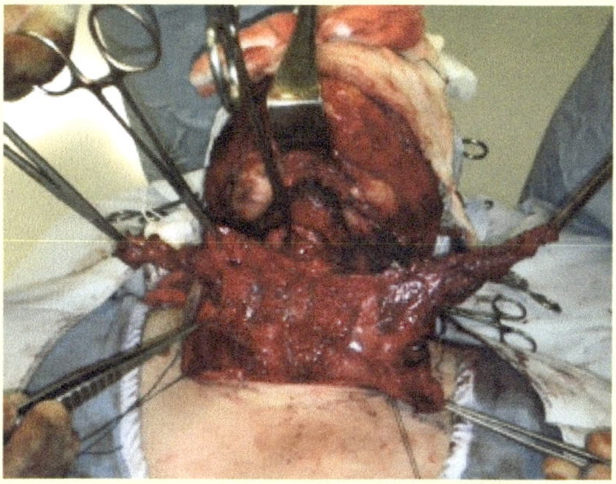

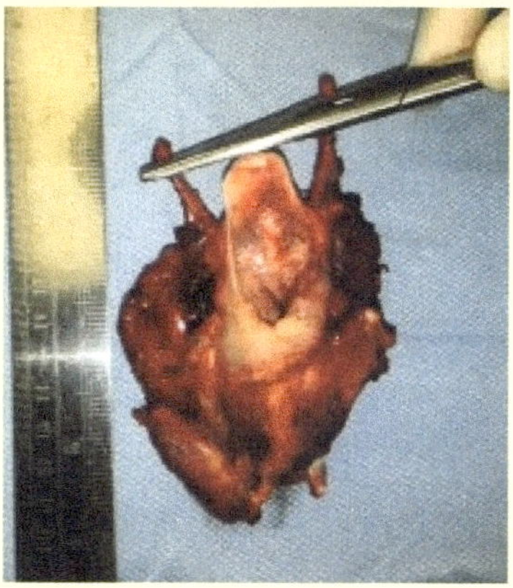

Figure 4.3.2 Picture of Laryngectomy and neck dissection for advance laryngeal cancer

Focusing question	Answer
What is a laryngectomy?	• Removal of larynx (partial vs total)
What are the indications?	• Laryngeal Cancer • Incompetent larynx, e.g. following radiotherapy
Can you name some of the complications?	• Immediate (≤24 hours post-op) o Primary Haemorrhage o Damage to surrounding structures: pneumothorax, chyle leak, hypoglossal nerve palsy • Early (1-14 days post-op) o Secondary haemorrhage o Pharyngocutaneous fistula • Late (> 14 days post-op) o Strictures (commonly cause dysphagia), dysphonia
What are the important factors to consider after laryngectomy?	Involve the Multi-Disciplinary Team • Speech Rehabilitation: o Tracheo-oesophageal puncture (TOP) ▪ Insertion of prosthesis o Oesophageal speech ▪ Air regurgitated through pharyngo-oesophageal segment to produce sound

	- Servox/Electrolarynx - External vibrating source • Stoma management • Specialist psychology input

4.3.3 RECONSTRUCTION IN THE HEAD AND NECK

Clinical Picture

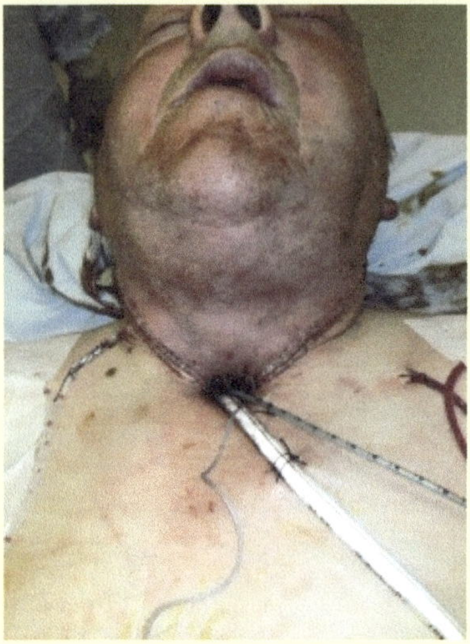

Figure 4.3.3 Neck reconstruction after laryngectomy

Focusing question	Answer
What are the different techniques used for reconstruction?	**1. Direct Closure** • Ideal for small defects **2. Skin graft** • Section of epidermis and dermis that has been removed from donor site: o Split skin graft: - Epidermis + Thin layer of dermis o Full-thickness - Epidermis + Full dermis

	3. Pedicled Flaps • Remain attached to their base allowing vascularity **4. Free Flap** • Bring own vasculature, however vascular anastomoses required through microsurgery **5. Prosthesis**
What is the difference between grafts and flaps?	**Grafts:** • Does not carry it's own vascular supply from the donor site, useful for smaller defects. **Flaps:** • Carries its blood supply, requires more extensive surgery but better outcomes for larger defects, or where recipient site is poorly vascularised.
What are the main types of flaps used for head & neck reconstruction?	**Pedicled. e.g.** • Pectoralis Major • Deltopectoral **Free flap. E.g.** • Jejunal • Antero-lateral thigh • Latissimus dorsi
What are the advantages of free flaps over pedicled flaps?	• Better function • Usually more tissue available and improved functional results • Reduced donor site morbidity if using a free flap.

What is the disadvantages of free flaps over pedicled flaps?	• More extensive surgery, often requires 2 teams (ENT + plastics) • Higher chance of flap failure
Can you name some of the possible contraindications to free flap reconstruction?	• Coagulopathies • Significant cardiac co-morbidities

Chapter 5

Paediatric Otolaryngology

5.1 CONGENITAL ABNORMALITIES

5.1.1 CONGENITAL ABNORMALITIES OF EARS AND HEARING

Clinical scenario

A 5-year-old child presents with his parents who are concerned with her hearing. She does not respond if his back is turned and his speech development is poor for his age. She does not have any other known medical problems but they believe his grandfather suffered from hearing problems at a young age. Her right ear is shown here (the left ear is the same).

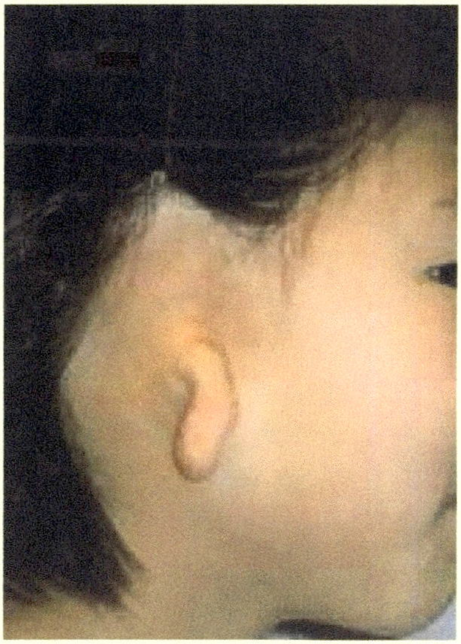

Figure 5.1.1 Microtia

<table>
<tr><th>Focusing question</th><th>Answer</th></tr>
<tr><td>How do you classify congenital hearing loss? Name some of the disorders.</td><td>Sensorineural
• Cochlear abnormalities, usually congenital
• Infective causes: Cytomegalovirus, rubella, toxoplasmosis
• Ototoxicity

Conductive
• Genetic disorders of external/middle ear
    o Microtia associated with external ear canal atresia
    o Fixed ossicles
• Genetic conditions associated with middle ear effusion
    o Down's syndrome
    o Cystic fibrosis
• Congenital cholesteatoma

Other rare syndromes which commonly appear in medical school exams and associations. All are associated with hearing loss.

• Pendred's syndrome - Thyroid goitre
• Usher's syndrome – Visual disturbance: retinitis pigmentosa
• Jervell Lang-Nielson syndrome – Cardiac arrhythmias: prolonged QT interval.
• Alport's syndrome – a disorder of type</td></tr>
</table>

<table>
<tr><td></td><td>4 collagen. Also presents with glomerulonephritis. (Causes a nephritic syndrome.)<ul><li>Neurofibromatosis (NF2) – Bilateral acoustic neuromas</li></ul></td></tr>
<tr><th>Management</th><th>Answer</th></tr>
<tr><td>What questions would you ask in this patient?</td><td><ul><li>Progressive hearing loss or present since birth?</li><li>Severity?</li><li>Developmental delay?</li><li>Past medical/family history?</li><li>Other medical problems- is this part of a syndrome?</li></ul></td></tr>
<tr><td>How would you examine this patient, and what would you look for?</td><td><ul><li>Full ENT, Head & Neck Examination: facial/ear deformities</li><li>Full paediatric examination: Syndromic features</li></ul></td></tr>
<tr><td>What possible investigations could you request for this patient?</td><td><ul><li>Basic hearing tests: PTA, Tympanometry</li><li>Specialist hearing tests: Otoacoustic emissions, brainstem evoked response audiometry</li></ul></td></tr>
<tr><td>How would you treat this patient?</td><td><ul><li>Specific ENT/audiology:<ul><li>Hearing aid/cochlear impants/bone-anchored hearing aid (BAHA)</li></ul></li><li>Supportive:</li></ul></td></tr>
</table>

	o Counselling/support o Referral to geneticist for gene testing
Additional Question (s)	**Answer**
What congenital abnormalities can affect the different parts of the ear?	**External Ear** • Anotia – lack of auricle • Microtia – underdeveloped auricle • Pre-auricular sinus- disorder of fusion of the hillocks that form the pinna. **External Ear Canal** • Stenosis • Atresia **Middle Ear** • Congenital malformations of ossicles **Inner-ear Malformations** • Cochlear aplasia - Cochlear fails to develop • Mondini's dysplasia. - Cochlear has one and one-half turns (normal = two and one-half turns)

5.1.2 CONGENITAL ABNORMALITIES OF THE NOSE

Clinical scenario
As the ENT SHO on-call, the paediatricians call you urgently as a child who has just been born through an emergency crash caesarean section is in respiratory distress. They suspect an upper airway cause. The mother reports that that one of her cousins may have had a similar problem at birth. On initial examination, you note that the child is in clear respiratory distress that seems to be relieved when she cries.

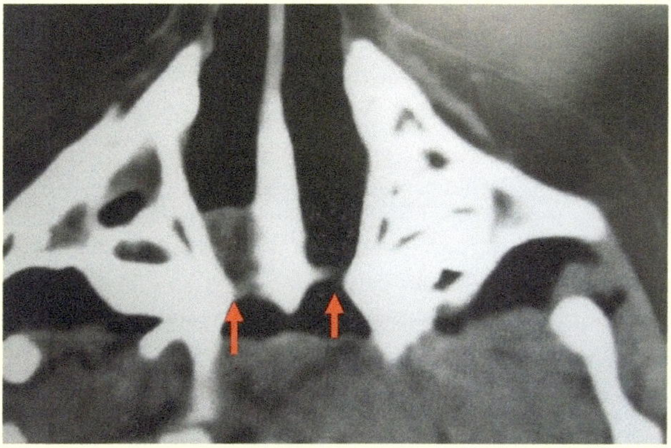

Figure 5.1.2 Axial CT Scan showing bilateral choanal atresia. *(Image from ENT Tzar Urgent Care in Otolaryngology)*

Focusing question	Answer
What is the most likely diagnosis?	Choanal atresia • Embryological abnormality (persistence) of bucconasal membrane. This covers the posterior aperture of the nasal cavity (choana).

<table>
<tr><td></td><td><ul><li>Associated with other congenital abnormalities in majority of conditions (Most common = CHARGE syndrome)</li></ul></td></tr>
<tr><td>How does this present?</td><td>Bilateral<ul><li>Respiratory distress in newborn</li><li>Neonates are almost completely dependent on nasal breathing</li><li>Partially relieved when baby cries (mouth opening helps relieve obstruction)</li></ul>Unilateral<ul><li>Presents later in life:<ul><li>Unilateral discharge/obstruction</li></ul></li></ul></td></tr>
<tr><th>Management</th><th>Answer</th></tr>
<tr><td>What is the management of bilateral choanal atresia?</td><td><ul><li>This is an airway emergency: call for senior support</li><li>Airway adjuncts (as nasal passages blocked, aim for inhalation through mouth)<ul><li>Oropharyngeal tube</li><li>Orotracheal intubation</li></ul></li><li>Investigations:<ul><li>Direct visualisation: FNE</li><li>Radiology: CT scan</li></ul></li><li>Treatment: Surgical.</li></ul></td></tr>
</table>

5.1.3 CONGENITAL ABNORMALITIES: CLEFT CONDITIONS

Clinical scenario
A pregnant lady has had an antenatal ultrasound scan and is told that her baby is very likely to have a cleft palate. She is concerned and her doctor has asked you to speak to her. She has a few questions.

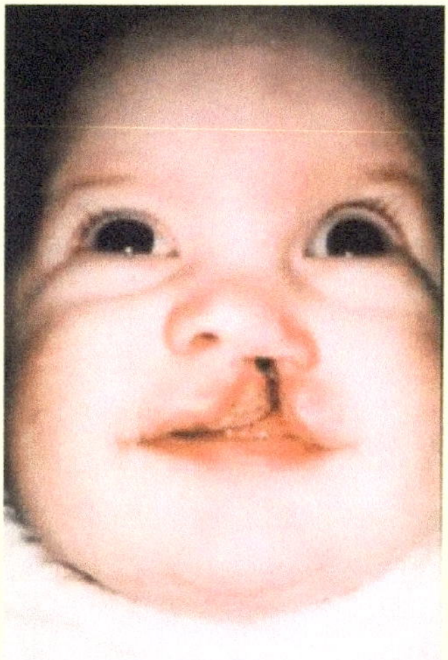

Figure 5.1.3: Unilateral cleft lip

Focusing question	Answer
What are the common cleft conditions?	**Cleft Lip** • Disruption in the development of muscles of upper lip and nasolabial region • Unilateral vs. bilateral **Cleft Palate** • Failure of fusion of the two palatine

	shelves • Cleft palate vs. submucous cleft palate (soft palate only)
Management	**Answer**

How is it managed?	• Multidisciplinary team.
	• Treated by surgical repair
	  o Cleft lip – one stage
	  o Cleft palate – one or two stage

Additional Question (s)	**Answer**
How can cleft lip/palate affect the ENT system?	**Hearing** • Conductive hearing loss – Eustachian tube dysfunction may result in OME • Sensorineural hearing loss – more common in syndromic cases **Airway** • Pierre Robin syndrome- characterised by micrognathism/retrognathism, retracted tongue, cleft palate – hypoxic episodes, particularly during feeding/sleeping **Speech** • Hypernasal speech (velopharyngeal insufficiency) • Dysarthria **Feeding** • Breast-feeding is difficult in some cases. **Dental anomalies** Orthodontist/Maxillofacial Surgery input may be required

5.1.4 CONGENITAL ABNORMALITIES OF THE NECK

Clinical scenario
A 5-year-old baby is brought in by his parents as they have noticed a lump in his neck, which his parents think is growing in size slowly. He is otherwise well. He has had a normal birth and normal developmental milestones. On examination he is well.

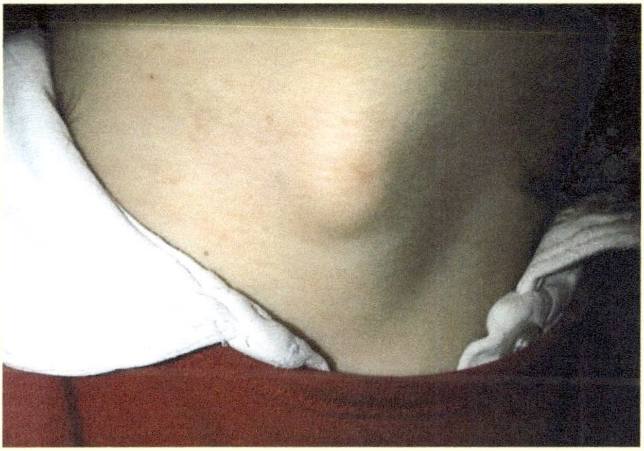

Figure 5.1.4 anterior neck lump (Thyroglossal duct cyst) in a child

Focusing question	Answer
What are the most common congenital/developmental neck lumps and how would you differentiate between them?	**Thyroglossal cyst** (refer to thyroid section) **Branchial cyst** • Embryological origin most commonly from 2nd branchial

<table>
<tr>
<td></td>
<td>
cleft
<ul>
<li>Usually present in early adulthood</li>
<li>Painless lump, usually at the anterior border of the sternocleidomastoid at junction of upper and middle thirds</li>
<li>Investigations:
<ul>
<li>FNA: “straw coloured” fluid containing cholesterol crystals</li>
<li>Ultrasound will confirm a cystic nature.</li>
<li>MRI can be useful to look for extension of the cyst into the neck.</li>
</ul>
</li>
<li>Management:
<ul>
<li>Aspiration. But high tendency to recur.</li>
<li>Surgery is preferred.</li>
</ul>
</li>
</ul>
Note: Can mimic malignant lymph node

Laryngocoele
<ul>
<li>Due to expansion of laryngeal saccule</li>
<li>Presentation: Intermittent soft neck swelling, voice hoarseness, stridor (can be asymptomatic)</li>
<li>O/E: Neck swelling on</li>
</ul>
</td>
</tr>
</table>

	palpation. If not palpable initially, becomes more evident on valsalva manoeuvre • Management: If symptomatic, surgical excision **Dermoid cyst** • At areas of embryological fusion e.g. lateral edge of eye brows. • Presentation: Painless lump • Management: Surgical excision **Carotid body tumour (Chemodectoma)** • Presentation: Painless lump often found at carotid bifurcation • More common geographically in areas of higher altitude. • Majority are benign, 10% malignant • O/E: Pulsatile mass. Classical moves laterally but not up and down. • Ix: Doppler US, CT, MRI, angiography. Do not try to aspirate or biopsy! • Mx: Surgical excision

Management	Answer
What questions would you ask?	• When did they first notice it: was it present at birth, or did it spontaneously appear? • How has it changed? • Is the child otherwise well? • Recent high temperature? • Family history? • Birth/developmental abnormalities?
How would you examine this patient?	• Full ENT examination including FNE if you suspect airway compression o Please refer to Examinations chapter for comprehensive examination of neck lumps. • Important to note position of lump in neck (be aware of the various triangles that the neck can be divided into)

How would you investigate the patient?	• Radiological:
	  o Ultrasound
	  o CT/MRI usually for more complex lumps
	• Fine Needle Aspiration

Outline the treatment options for the patient	• Conservative • Surgical excision

5.2 GENETIC SYNDROMES

5.2.1 DOWN'S SYNDROME AND ENT

Clinical scenario
A pregnant 37 year old sees you as she is seeking advice concerning her child. Following antenatal testing for Down's syndrome screening, the lady received diagnostic intervention by way of amniocentesis. The results revealed a chance that the foetus may have Down's syndrome. She approaches you with several questions.

Focusing question	Answer
What is it caused by?	• Trisomy 21 • Affects 1/700 births
Additional Question (s)	**Answer**
Can you name some of the ENT features of Down's syndrome?	**Ear** • Conductive hearing loss – otitis media with effusion • Sensorineural hearing loss • Low-set pinna • Narrow external ear canals – increased risk of otitis externa **Nose** • Low nasal bridge **Throat** • Macroglossia • Narrow pharynx • Subglottic stenosis

5.2.2 OTHER SYNDROMES AND ENT

Syndromes	Features
Velo-cardio-facial syndrome	• Autosomal dominant – abnormality affecting chromosome 22q11 • ENT features: o Ear: Conductive hearing loss o Nose: Prominent nose Facial features: Narrow palpebral fissures
Treacher-Collins syndrome	• Autosomal dominant, at least 50% sporadic • ENT features: o Ear: Microtia, ossicular malformation o Nose: "Bird face" deformity o Throat: Cleft palate • Facial features: o Maxillary and mandibular hypoplasia
Goldenhar Syndrome	• Most common due to sporadic mutations • ENT features: o Ear: Microtia, canal atresia o Throat: Cleft lip/palate, velopharyngeal incompetence • Facial features: o Facial asymmetry o Mandibular hypoplasia • Very similar features to Treacher-Collins syndrome. However, some patients with Goldenhar show signs of mental retardation as opposed to Treacher Collins.

CHARGE Syndrome	• Common features: o **C**oloboma o **H**eart Defects o Choanal **A**tresia o Growth **R**etardation o **G**enitourinary malformations o **E**ar abnormalities

5.3 PAEDIATRIC AIRWAYS

5.3.1 PAEDIATRIC AIRWAY ISSUES

Clinical scenario

A 4 year old child is brought into the A&E department by his parents with noisy breathing and obvious respiratory distress. He has had normal developmental milestones. On further questioning, his parents report that he has recently had a high temperature and a cough. On examination, you note that he is drooling. His chest is clear, however there is marked intercostal recession and tracheal tug.

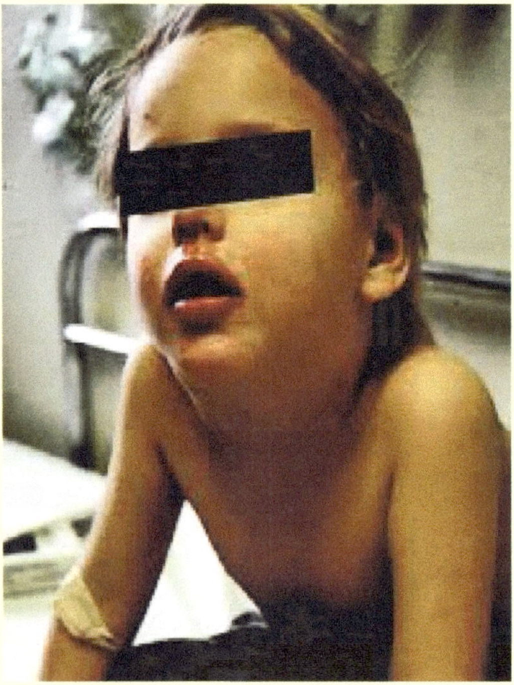

Figure 5.3.1a Child adoping the tripod position typical of epiglottis

Focusing question	Answer
Can you name some causes of airway obstruction in children?	**Infective** • Croup • Epiglottitis • Severe tonsillitis • Parapharyngeal abscess **Congenital** • Laryngomalacia- commonest cause of stridor in children. • Subglottic stenosis
Management	**Answer**
What questions would you ask in the history?	(Refer to adult airway obstruction for more comprehensive management) • Previous episodes • Recent lower or upper respiratory tract infection • Possibility of inhalation of foreign body, e.g. unilateral nasal discharge • Neonatal intubation or time in intensive care. Can predispose to tracheal stenosis. • Past medical history, developmental milestones • Vaccination history. Consider epiglottitis in patients not vaccinated with HIB vaccine • Family history of ENT/airway problems

<table>
<tr><td>How would you examine the patient?</td><td>Do NOT distress children, especially if you suspect epiglottitis, as this may compromise the airway

<ul>
<li>Look:
<ul>
<li>Respiratory distress: increased respiratory rate, use of accessory muscles, intercostal recession, tracheal tug, cyanosis</li>
<li>Full ENT examination including FNE to determine potential cause of obstruction, including foreign body.</li>
</ul></li>
<li>Listen:
<ul>
<li>Stridor (noisy breathing due to laryngeal or tracheal obstruction)</li>
<li>Stertor (noisy breathing due to supra-laryngeal obstruction)</li>
</ul></li>
<li>Pyrexia</li>
</ul></td></tr>
<tr><td>How would you treat the patient?</td><td>This is a potential emergency, if in doubt put out an emergency call early – you would need anaesthetic, ENT and paediatric support
<ul>
<li>Maintain own airway:
<ul>
<li>Humidified oxygen</li>
<li>Nebulised adrenaline (reduces mucosal oedema)</li>
<li>Heliox (less dense that oxygen alone)</li>
<li>Dexamethasone (reduces airway oedema)</li>
</ul></li>
<li>Airway Manoeuvres:
<ul>
<li>Positioning: Neutral, Sniffing the morning air or Jaw Thrust</li>
</ul></li>
</ul></td></tr>
</table>

<table>
<tr><td></td><td>

- Airway adjuncts:
  - Nasopharyngeal airway
  - Oropharyngeal airway
- Intubation/Laryngeal Mask Airway
  - Surgical airway – Cricothyroidotomy/Tracheostomy (always a last resort)

</td></tr>
<tr><th>Additional Question (s)</th><th>Answer</th></tr>
<tr><td>What are the main differences between a paediatric and adult airway?</td><td>

- Larger oropharyngeal soft tissues (tongue and tonsils) relatively compared to adults.
  - Increased likelihood to obstruct airway
  - Difficult visualisation
- The smaller the child, larger cranium compared to the midface, i.e. Larger occiput
  - Affects head positioning - use neutral position in youngest children
- Narrow funnel-shaped airway
- Short trachea (infant: 5cm)
  - Easier to accidentally intubate right main bronchus

</td></tr>
<tr><td>How could you differentiate between the different causes of airways</td><td>

Croup (laryngotracheobronchitis)

- PC: Inspiratory stridor + harsh barking cough
- Usually associated with URTI
- Affects children aged from 6 months to 4 years (younger vs epiglottitis)
- Due to inflammatory oedema in

</td></tr>
</table>

obstruction?	subglottic region (this is already the narrowest part of paediatric airway)
	• Usually self-limiting
	• Mx: Oxygen, antibiotics, dexamethasone
	• If deteriorates, intubation (rarely necessary)
	
	Epiglottitis
	• Aetiology: Haemophilus influenzae type B commonest. Therefore you must ask about the vaccination history.
	• Usually affects children 2-6 years old (older vs croup)
	• Associated with URTI, shorter history than croup, child looks more unwell
	• PC: Inspiratory stridor, pyrexia, drooling
	  o Child usually leans forward, drooling
	• ***Management:***
	  o Do **not** examine if this would cause distress, as this may compromise the airway
	  o Call for senior anaesthetic and ENT support **early**
	  o The child will maintain upright posture as this is most comfortable
	  o Move child to safe area (theatre) with anaesthetic support – intubation if required.
	  o Anaesthetist to perform direct laryngoscopy, in a controlled safe environment to identify inflamed swollen epiglottis

- Intubate if possible (rigid ventilating bronchoscope may be helpful), otherwise emergency tracheostomy
- Once airway safeguarded, IV antibiotics, humidified oxygen
- Once child is well, usually after 48 hours, attempt extubation

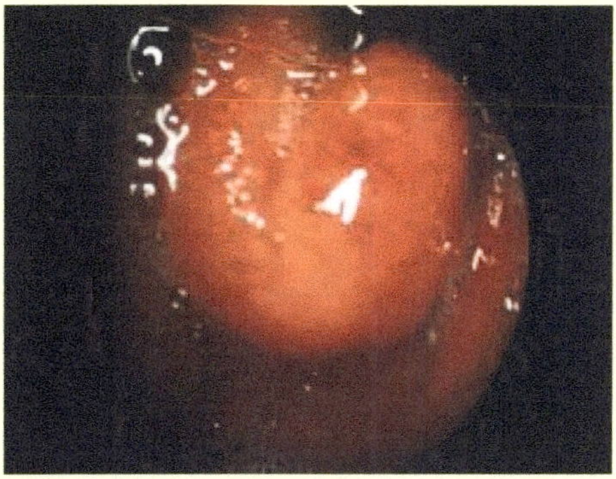

Figure 5.3.1b Swollen epiglottis typical of epiglottis

Laryngomalacia

- Due to floppy arytenoids and aryepiglottic folds that collapse during inspiration.
- Usually presents very shortly after birth
- Associated with reflux disease, but the direction of causality is unclear.
- Commonest cause of paediatric stridor
- Management:
    - Conservative in the majority of cases: Generally symptoms will

	settle within 18 months as the cartilage matures. Reflux medications may be of benefit. o Surgery (rarely required): laryngoscopy & aryepiglottoplasty **Subglottic stenosis** • Subglottis = narrowest section of paediatric airway • Presentation: Stridor, recurrent episodes of croup • Risk factors: o Recurrent/Prolonged intubation o Laryngopharyngeal reflux • Mx: o Initial airway management o If mild: endoscopic dilatation o If severe: ▪ Tracheostomy and follow-up. If lumen increasing in size during growth, tracheostomy can be removed. ▪ Surgery: Laryngotracheoplasty (reconstructive surgery)

5.3.2 OBSTRUCTIVE SLEEP APNOEA

Clinical scenario
A 4 year old child has been referred to your ENT clinic by his GP. His parents are concerned about his breathing, which is particularly noisy at night. They feel that there are periods when he stops breathing, and this waked him up at night. He has been irritable and concentrates poorly during the day. Examination revealed large tonsils.

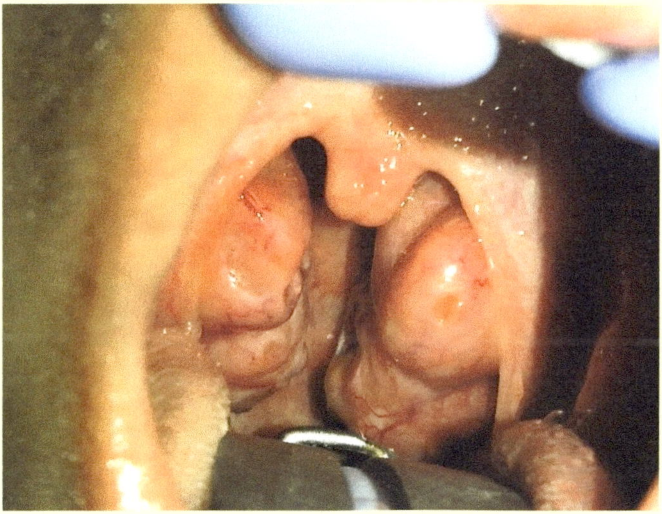

Figure 5.3.2 : Huge tonsils blocking more that 75% of the oropharyngeal airway (Grade IV)

Focusing question	Answer
What is the differential diagnosis?	• Obstructive sleep apnoea (OSA) • Habitual snoring

Management	Answer

How could you investigate this patient?	(Please refer to adult airway obstruction for more comprehensive management)
	• Full ENT exam, including FNE to look for any obvious causes of obstruction
	• Sleep study – polysomnography.
	  o Children:
	    ▪ Apnoea Hypopnoea Index (AHI) > 5 events per hour = indication for treatment
	  o Adults:
	    ▪ AHI < 5 = normal
	    ▪ AHI 5 -15 = mild
	    ▪ AHI 15 - 30 = moderate
	    ▪ AHI > 30 = severe

How would you treat this patient?	Children
	• Conservative:
	  o Weight loss if overweight
	• Medical:
	  o Continuous positive airway pressure
	• Surgical:
	  o Adenotonsillectomy – most common cause of OSA in children (this would need to be done in a specialist paediatric centre)
	
	Adults
	• Conservative:
	  o Weight loss, Stop smoking, Stop alcohol
	  o Mandibular advancement

	devices/splints
	• Medical:
	  o Continuous positive airway pressure
	• Surgical (dependent on cause):
	  o Adenotonsillectomy
	  o Nasal turbinectomy
	  o Uvuloplatopharyngoplasty (UPPP)
	  o Mandibular advancement

Additional Question (s)	**Answer**
What are the causes of obstructive sleep apnoea?	Children: • Adenotonsillar enlargement (most common reason) • Obesity • Syndrome Adults: • Overweight/obesity – large neck • Long uvula/small jaw

Other publications by the ENTTZAR TEAM

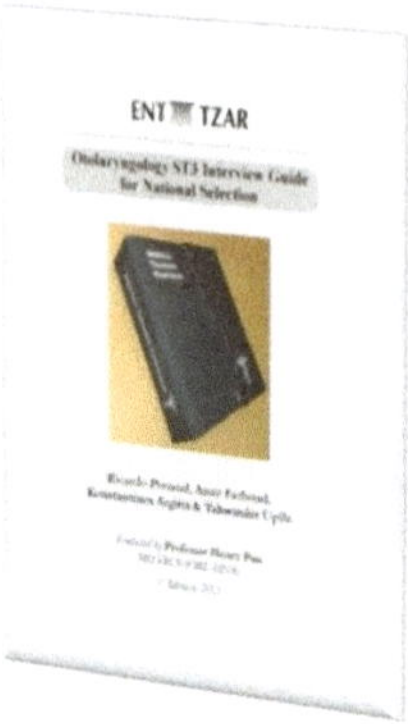

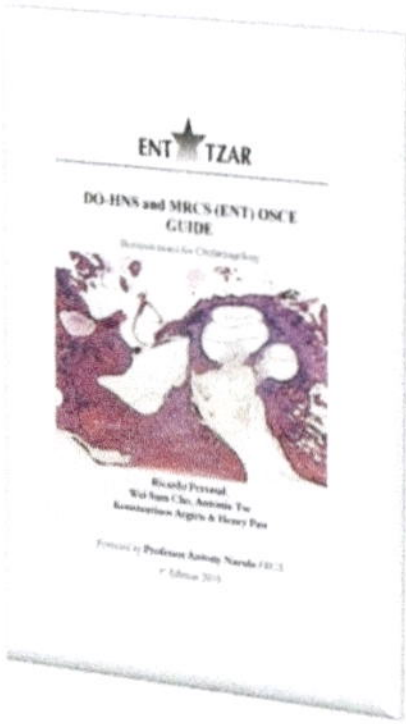

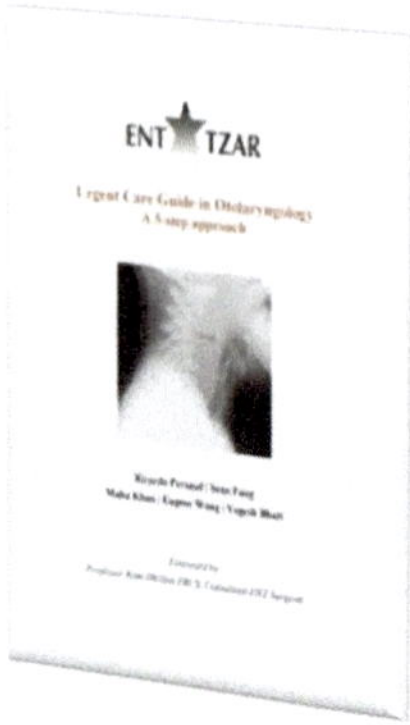

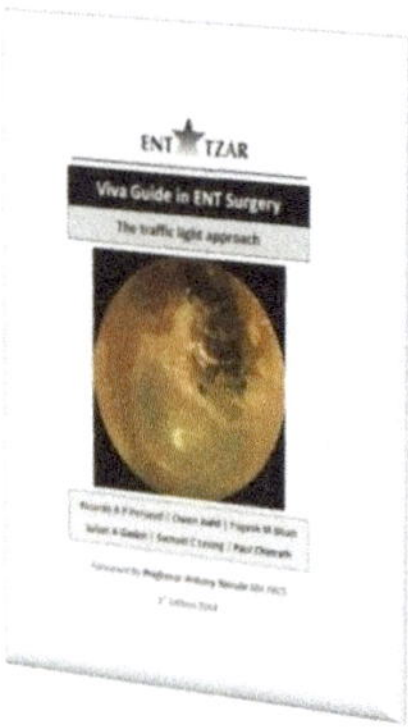

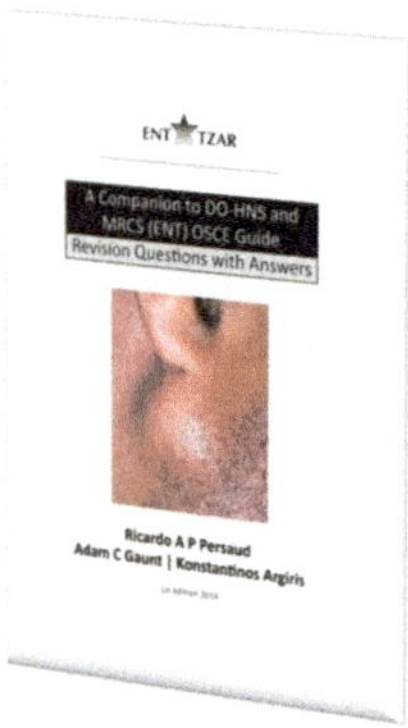

* 9 7 8 1 7 8 4 5 6 1 7 1 0 *

ND - #0107 - 060826 - C250 - 197/132/14 - PB - 9781784561710 - Gloss Lamination